Harm Reduction Approaches with Adolescents Who Use Substances

Harm Reduction Approaches with Adolescents Who Use Substances details the concepts of harm reduction and how they can be implemented in work with adolescents on the topic of substance use behaviors.

This book reviews the concepts of harm reduction as they have traditionally been applied and in the context of working with adolescents around issues of substance use behaviors. Using both conceptual and real-world examples, this book guides students through case examples and exercises designed to not only better understand harm reduction as a concept, but to practice putting it to use in real world clinical scenarios. This book also aims to reduce the stigma associated with talking about substance-using behavior and to provide nuance around different types of use, from experimental to hazardous, using person-first language without resorting to shaming and blaming. Practical elements incorporate skills of Motivational Interviewing (MI) and Cognitive Behavioral Therapy (CBT) into discussion.

Suitable for use in a variety of upper-level and graduate courses, this book educates students about the traditional concepts of harm reduction and how they can relate to adolescent substance use and family therapy.

Amanda Reiman, Ph.D., MSW, is a public health researcher who has been studying cannabis as a harm reduction tool for 20+ years. She is the founder of Personal Plants, an education platform focused on helping people develop healthy, balanced relationships with cannabis. In development is a 10-week online program called Cannabis in Balance which helps people identify and change unhealthy behaviors around cannabis use. Dr. Reiman earned her Ph.D. in Social Welfare from the University of California, Berkeley, and conducted one of the first research studies on medical cannabis patients and the use of cannabis as a substitute for alcohol and other drugs. She then taught courses on substance abuse, drug policy, and sexuality at Berkeley for 11 years. Dr. Reiman is an internationally recognized cannabis expert and public health researcher. Formerly the in-house cannabis expert for the Drug Policy Alliance, she has written for and has been quoted in numerous national and international publications as well as peer reviewed academic journals and several textbooks. Dr. Reiman currently lives just outside of Tacoma, Washington, with her partner, Sean, and their two cats and two dogs.

Barry Lessin, M.Ed., CAADC, is a harm reduction psychologist in private practice, specializing in working with individuals and families impacted by substance use. With a career spanning nearly 50 years, Barry has served as a clinician, drug policy advocate, educator, researcher, and administrator. He has experience providing services across the entire continuum of addiction treatment, and draws on an integrative approach informed by decades of work across intersecting systems – mental health, substance use treatment, and grassroots policy reform. His work has been informed by program development and oversight roles at innovative addiction treatment centers, including serving as Director of the first substance use program integrated into a community mental health center in Philadelphia, and contributing to the development of the city's first intensive outpatient addiction treatment program. Over the past 15 years, his focus shifted to drug policy reform and family advocacy, where he collaborated with harm reduction pioneers and held clinical leadership and capacity-building roles in nonprofit organizations to expand access to harm reduction education and treatment for families facing systemic barriers to care. Barry played an important role in a grassroots coalition that advanced Pennsylvania's 911 Good Samaritan and naloxone access legislation – vital public health measures that provide legal protections during overdose emergencies and expand access to lifesaving naloxone. He currently lives in suburban Philadelphia with his wife, Jennifer, and two cats.

"This is a book that will lower parental anxieties and help teens engage in honest conversations about drug use. Lessin and Reiman have taken science and clinical wisdom to develop their IDEA structure – a collaborative conversation that places the complexity of teen drug use in the context of normal adolescent development."

Patt Denning, *Ph.D., Director of Clinical Services and Training at the Harm Reduction Therapy Center, co-author of* Practicing Harm Reduction Psychotherapy: An Alternative Approach to Addictions

"In their new book, *Harm Reduction Approaches with Adolescents Who Use Substances*, Barry Lessin and Amanda Reiman are on the cutting edge of new thinking about working with adolescents. Called harm reduction, this approach has the following defining characteristics: 1) adolescents are treated with respect as collaborators in the change and healing process; 2) use of substances by young people is not entirely ruled out, nor taken as a sign of an irresolvable, lifelong disease. Rather, the entire child, their outlook and relationships with the people and the world around them, are the building blocks for the Lessin-Reiman adolescent helping approach. If their approach sounds like plain common sense, steeped in what readers understand to be the basics of sound parenting and youth development – so be it. For Lessin and Reiman there can be no better sign that they are tracking with the best practices for yielding healthy functioning at any age."

Stanton Peele, *Ph.D., founder, Life Process Program for Addiction Coaching, author of* A Scientific Life on the Edge: My Lonely Quest to Change How We See Addiction

"This book finally provides the much-needed response to the question that harm reductionists are asked every day: "But what about the kids?" In this comprehensive book, Reiman and Lessin provide families, providers, and communities with a framework with which to understand why young people use drugs and how to support them to make safer choices."

Sheila P. Vakharia, *Ph.D., MSW, author of* The Harm Reduction Gap

Harm Reduction Approaches with Adolescents Who Use Substances

Amanda Reiman and Barry Lessin

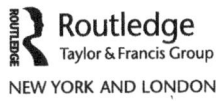

NEW YORK AND LONDON

Designed cover image: Getty Images

First published 2026
by Routledge
605 Third Avenue, New York, NY 10158

and by Routledge
4 Park Square, Milton Park, Abingdon, Oxon, OX14 4RN

Routledge is an imprint of the Taylor & Francis Group, an informa business

© 2026 Amanda Reiman and Barry Lessin

The right of Amanda Reiman and Barry Lessin to be identified as authors of this work has been asserted in accordance with sections 77 and 78 of the Copyright, Designs and Patents Act 1988.

All rights reserved. No part of this book may be reprinted or reproduced or utilised in any form or by any electronic, mechanical, or other means, now known or hereafter invented, including photocopying and recording, or in any information storage or retrieval system, without permission in writing from the publishers.

For Product Safety Concerns and Information please contact our EU representative GPSR@taylorandfrancis.com. Taylor & Francis Verlag GmbH, Kaufingerstraße 24, 80331 München, Germany.

Trademark notice: Product or corporate names may be trademarks or registered trademarks, and are used only for identification and explanation without intent to infringe.

Library of Congress Cataloging-in-Publication Data
Names: Reiman, Amanda author | Lessin, Barry author
Title: Harm reduction approaches with adolescents who use substances / Amanda Reiman and Barry Lessin.
Description: New York, NY : Routledge, 2026. | Includes bibliographical references and index. |
Contents: Harm reduction history and concepts -- Examples of harm reduction in the current substance use landscape -- Drug using behavior in adolescence -- Substance use in adolescence: potential harms and suggested approaches -- Drug policy's impact on addiction treatment and drug education -- Key considerations in practicing HRT -- Core dilemmas in practicing harm reduction therapy -- Essentials of adolescent development and parenting -- Why HRT works well with adolescents -- Adolescent HRT in practice -- Trauma-informed care -- Working with parents -- Exercises.
Identifiers: LCCN 2025026468 (print) | LCCN 2025026469 (ebook) | ISBN 9781032948263 hbk | ISBN 9781032940847 pbk | ISBN 9781003581857 ebk
Subjects: LCSH: Teenagers -- Substance use | Substance abuse -- Treatment | Harm reduction
Classification: LCC RJ506.D78 R435 2026 (print) | LCC RJ506.D78 (ebook)
LC record available at https://lccn.loc.gov/2025026468
LC ebook record available at https://lccn.loc.gov/2025026469

ISBN: 978-1-032-94826-3 (hbk)
ISBN: 978-1-032-94084-7 (pbk)
ISBN: 978-1-003-58185-7 (ebk)

DOI: 10.4324/9781003581857

Typeset in Times New Roman
by SPi Technologies India Pvt Ltd (Straive)

Dr. Amanda Reiman would like to dedicate this book to the pioneers of harm reduction. The advocates, policy makers, and educators who have championed this approach in the face of backlash. And especially the population of people who use drugs, and their tireless fight for visibility, humanity, and safer lives.

Barry Lessin would like to dedicate this book to the families and parent advocates I've learned from – those who have supported adolescents through substance use, emotional challenges, and systems that have too often let them down. Your persistence and resilience has shaped the way I approach this work. I also want to acknowledge the professionals and educators who are working to expand access to care that is respectful, practical, and developmentally appropriate. Your efforts continue to move the field forward. This book is intended as a resource for all of you – and for the young people at the center of this work.

Contents

Preface   *xi*

PART I
Welcome to Harm Reduction   1
AMANDA REIMAN PH.D., MSW

1 Harm Reduction History and Concepts   5

2 Examples of Harm Reduction in the Current Substance Use Landscape   11

3 Drug Using Behavior in Adolescence   17

4 Substance Use in Adolescence: Potential Harms and Suggested Approaches   25

5 Drug Policy's Impact on Addiction Treatment and Drug Education   39

PART II
Addressing Substance Use with Harm Reduction Treatment Strategies   51
BARRY LESSIN M.ED., CAADC

6 Key Considerations in Practicing HRT   55

7 Core Dilemmas in Practicing Harm Reduction Therapy   60

8 Essentials of Adolescent Development and Parenting   73

9 Why HRT Works Well with Adolescents   86

10 Adolescent HRT in Practice   97

11 Trauma-Informed Care   115

12	Working with Parents	120
13	Exercises	135
	Conclusion and Key Takeaways	147

Appendix A   *151*
Appendix B   *152*
Bibliography   *155*
Index   *166*

Preface

This book is for anyone with a stake in adolescent well-being: current and aspiring therapists, school counselors, healthcare providers, educators, and caregivers. Whether you do or will sit with teens in clinics, classrooms, living rooms, or community programs, the work of supporting young people is complex – and often urgent. Substance use, emotional distress, school pushout, and system involvement don't show up in isolation. They are entangled with identity development, peer dynamics, intergenerational trauma, family stress, and structural inequities.

Mainstream models of adolescent substance use treatment have too often prioritized abstinence, compliance, and diagnosis over understanding, context, and relationship. These models frequently overlook the ways in which substance use can function – for regulation, connection, escape, identity formation – and fail to account for the developmental tasks adolescents are still navigating. And while families are essential to supporting youth, many have been left without clear guidance, appropriate support, or access to evidence-based care.

Harm reduction offers another path forward. It is not a soft alternative to "real" treatment – it is a rigorous, ethical, and relational approach that begins with respect: respect for autonomy, for ambivalence, for lived experience, and for the protective functions behaviors may serve. It centers safety, collaboration, and incremental change. It recognizes that the goal isn't to control behavior – it's to build trust, reduce harm, and support development in the real world as it is, not as we wish it were.

This book is grounded in that philosophy. We build on the foundational work of harm reduction pioneers such as Alan Marlatt, Patt Denning, Jeannie Little, Andrew Tatarsky, Stanton Peele and Scott Kellogg – each of whom challenged the moralism, rigidity, and false binaries of conventional substance use treatment. We've adapted their insights for the evolving needs of adolescents and for the adults – both professional and familial – working to support them.

Our perspective is also shaped by our work as drug policy advocates, focused on undoing the legacy of the War on Drugs. We have seen how criminalization, surveillance, and stigma have fractured families, denied people care, and turned adolescence into a high-stakes battleground. Families have not failed treatment – treatment has failed families by offering narrow, one-size-fits-all models that do not reflect the realities of young people's lives.

This book is dedicated to those families. To those who have experienced loss, stigma, and systemic exclusion – not because they didn't care, but because they weren't given real options. Their persistence, advocacy, and refusal to give up continue to shape the direction of this work.

We also write this book for the next generation of clinicians, educators, and helpers – those entering the field with a commitment to showing up for young people with integrity and clarity. We offer strategies that integrate harm reduction principles with developmentally responsive applications of Motivational Interviewing (MI), Cognitive Behavioral Therapy (CBT), Dialectical Behavior Therapy (DBT), and CRAFT (Community Reinforcement and Family Training). These approaches are not presented as protocols to follow, but as tools to be used with flexibility, curiosity, and respect.

Many say that engaging with adolescents can feel like a burden, but we view it as a privilege. It is exciting and humbling to witness a young person struggle, reflect, take risks, and discover who they are becoming. This book is a contribution to the ongoing effort to make that work more humane, more just, and more attuned to the realities of adolescence. We hope it supports your practice, affirms your instincts, and helps grow a future where care is centered not in fear, but in relationship.

Part I

Welcome to Harm Reduction

Amanda Reiman Ph.D., MSW

Welcome to Harm Reduction

Why did we write this book?

Talking about drug use is difficult. Not only are there real mental and physical health outcomes at stake, our society has attached mortality to the use of illicit substances (Duster, 1970; Peele, 1998). People who use drugs are often viewed as mentally ill, weak, lazy, and out of control. The United States has not only bought into the message that those who use drugs are "less than", we have gone so far as to say that people who use drugs are criminals. Drug offenses account for a significant portion of the federal prison population. As of recent reports, approximately 45% of federal inmates are incarcerated for drug-related offenses, equating to about 60,000–65,000 individuals. In state prisons, the percentage of individuals incarcerated for drug offenses is smaller compared to violence or property crimes. Drug offenses account for about 15–20% of state prisoners, translating to roughly 200,000–250,000 individuals annually. Many people are held in local jails on drug charges, often pretrial or for short sentences. On an annual basis, several hundred thousand individuals may cycle through jails for drug-related offenses, with some estimates ranging from 400,000–500,000 admissions. Annually, around 650,000–750,000 adults may be incarcerated (including federal, state, and local facilities) for drug-related charges, though this number can vary based on law enforcement practices, sentencing laws, and reforms like decriminalization or diversion programs (Department of Justice, 2024). This sends the message that people who use drugs are dangerous to society and must be kept separate from them. It also suggests that using drugs is an easy way to ruin your future and condemn you to a lifetime of criminal justice involvement. After all, those convicted of felony drug crimes continue to experience punishment after they are released from prison. Collateral sanctions for drug offenses can include the inability to vote, receive federal funding for college or access to public housing, obtain employment or a professional license, and adopt a child (Kimball & Grawert, 2021). And while 80% of people who use illicit substances do not enter addiction, the belief spouted from anti-drug propaganda is that even one time will get you "hooked" (Hart, 2021).

Because of the societal framing of drug use, the impact that a drug charge can have on your present and future, and the belief that drug addiction happens to 100% of drug users, it is no wonder that parents and educators feel that they must prevent teen substance use at all costs. To be clear, intoxicating substances of any kind, including alcohol and non-prescribed pharmaceutical drugs, are not appropriate for teens for reasons we will discuss. However, the going strategy has been to deploy the same basic tactics used on adult substance users to teens who are caught using drugs. Punishment, mandating traditional treatment, denial of privileges, detainment, and shaming are common current methods for deterring teen substance use. But we feel that there is a better way, rooted in public health and safety, and sensitive to the teen experience and family dynamics: harm reduction. (For the sake of consistency, we will use the term "traditional treatment" to refer to one-size-fits-all, abstinence-only models.)

There are four main reasons that we decided to write this book.

1. *To acknowledge the current "Just Say No" approach and the difficulty parents have with honest, pragmatic, and safety-based conversations with their teens about substance use.*

As we mentioned, drug users are framed as dangerous people with no future. There is also the belief that everyone who uses an illicit drug becomes addicted to it. Those who care about young people think that simply telling them not to use drugs because they are dangerous and addictive is enough. Unfortunately for them, developmental related impulses in teenagers sometimes make rational decision making a problem, and desire to be accepted by peers can influence behavior in ways that will not exist in adulthood. Looking at the data on teen substance use is enough to know that, while rare, teens ARE using drugs. In 2023, 6.5%, 11.3%, and 19.8% of 8th, 10th, and 12th graders, respectively, reported using an illicit drug in the past 30 days (Monitoring the Future, 2023). If we can accept that teen drug use happens, we should also acknowledge the failure of an abstinence only approach and the need for conversations about drugs that revolve around support and safety.

2. *To teach students about the traditional concepts of harm reduction and how they can be related to adolescent substance use and family therapy.*

Family systems theory tells us that the family is a connected web of established roles and ways of communicating that predict its functionality (McGinnis & Wright, 2023). Family therapy often focuses on these roles and connections as a way of detangling maladaptive patterns. When a teen in the family is using substances, regardless of whether that is a problem in and of itself, it can be disruptive to the system. Using techniques from the field of harm reduction can minimize the ripples caused by the substance use and instead invite the conversation about underlying factors without blame and judgment. The substance use itself should not be viewed as the cause of the rift, it is a warning sign that a rift exists and must be addressed. We explore this concept later in the book by examining the CRAFT method.

3. *To differentiate between experimentation and problematic use in the context of potential harms for all adolescent use of drugs and alcohol. And to also recognize the risks of drug and alcohol use during this time of personal development.*

"All use is abuse." This is a common trope in the discussions about drug use and addiction, fueled by the War on Drugs, abstinence-only treatment programs, and the Just Say No programs of the 1980s and 1990s. Interestingly, this claim only seems to apply to those who use illicit substances, as most of us know plenty of people who drink alcohol only occasionally and without incident. But, when it comes to adolescents, there is a zero tolerance policy for both alcohol and illicit drugs, as we will explore later in this book. But is it warranted? Should the same approach, for example, be taken with a kid who is doing well in school, has good relationships with his family, and close, supportive friends but gets caught smoking a joint in a park on a Saturday, and a kid who is having behavioral issues at school, trouble at home, and is getting drunk every morning before cutting class? The point is, that for everyone, including teens, all use is NOT abuse. Furthermore, all use is not the same and does warrant the same approach. We want to present a spectrum of substance use for adolescents that can guide a pragmatic and realistic response.

As previously mentioned, intoxicating substances of any kind not prescribed by their doctor are not appropriate for adolescents. Not only are adolescent brains still forming and developing, the developmental issues around behavior and risk taking mentioned earlier deem them not mature enough to always make rational decisions about drugs and alcohol. There is a reason we don't let teens drive until they are 16, vote when they are 18, and buy alcohol and cannabis (in legal markets) until they are 21. We are saying that their minds and bodies have not matured to a place where we can count on them to make sound and smart decisions about risky behaviors. Some may argue that kids should be able to buy alcohol at 18 since they are already finding ways to obtain it. But the point is that we restrict certain activities because of the risks of an immature and less developed approach to the behavior. But while we can acknowledge the risks of teen substance use, we have already established that it exists, even if we wish all teens abstained until they were old enough to handle the behavior responsibly.

4. *To allow students to practice what can sometimes be difficult discussions with parents and teens around this highly charged, emotional issue.*

By now it should be evident that approaching the topic of teen substance use with parents and families can be emotionally intense and met with fear. This fear of THEIR children succumbing to drug addiction and all of the societal scarlet letters that come with it can encourage them to take the antiquated "Just Say No" approach. And while a harm reduction approach is much more likely to keep their teen safe and encourage open and honest communication, doing anything but admonishing and punishing substance use feels like they are giving their teen a pass to use drugs. In this book you will find exercises that will allow you to practice the harm reduction approach, as well as the conversations you may have with parents concerned about their teen. These conversations may not be easy, but practicing them and learning more about harm reduction will up your skill level and confidence.

Chapter 1

Harm Reduction History and Concepts

Harm Reduction: History and Concepts

History

In this book, we are discussing harm reduction in the context of adolescent substance use. And while harm reduction has not always been centered on the issue of substance use, it has always been related to public health and personal safety, and rooted in compassion and activism. Programs that feed those who cannot afford food without passing judgment or asking for anything in return. Providing people who use drugs with access to alternative health and wellness treatments. Safe access to health services like abortion. These services and programs follow the concepts of harm reduction (National Harm Reduction Coalition, 2024: https://harmreduction.org/movement/evolution/). The public health crisis of HIV/AIDS in the 1980s is what sped up the evolution of harm reduction. The spread of HIV/AIDS was like a steam engine racing through the gay community as well as the community of people who used intravenous drugs. At the time, these communities were blamed for the spread, with talk centering around their moral choices. Some even thought that HIV/AIDS was a punishment for their lifestyles. As we later discovered (not soon enough to prevent the decimation of entire enclaves of people), the reason these communities were hit especially hard was because of the ways in which HIV/AIDS was contracted: through the exchange of blood and/or sexual fluids. Harm reduction seeks to provide strategies for making behaviors safer, without demanding that the behavior cease. In this case, providing condoms and clean needle kits. Without judgment. The message was simple. We do not want you to die. Using these safety tools will help you live (O'Hare, 2007). And thus, the concept of harm reduction places survival and good health above morally driven demands of abstinence. But harm reduction does not downplay or ignore the risks associated with sexual activity or substance use. Rather, harm reduction believes that there are ways to help people live healthier, longer lives, EVEN IF they continue to use substances (Marlatt, 1996).

One of the first places to implement a harm reduction approach to substance use was in Merseyside, United Kingdom, in response to heroin use. Relying on the framework of the old British system, the clinic in Merseyside reasoned that, for some people, heroin maintenance might be necessary to successfully treat them for other mental and physical health issues and for them to live a valuable life. Today, patients in Merseyside are still prescribed injectable heroin. Merseyside also started one of the first syringe exchange programs and gave their clients access to fresh food, knowing the importance of nutrition on physical and mental health. The program also had the support of local police, which helped remove criminal justice sanctions from the environment (Inciardi, 2000). In 1985, the Mersey Drug Training and

Information Center (MDTIC) opened. Next door to the Liverpool Drug Dependency Unit (LDDU), the MDTIC had a mission to provide public health-based, safety-focused information about drug use to anyone who wanted it and to train public health professionals on how to approach substance use and people who use drugs from a harm reduction perspective (O'Hare, 2007).

The idea of providing those who are drug dependent their drug of choice to stave off withdrawals and help them maintain a productive life used to be the law of the land in the United States. Up until the Harrison Narcotics Act of 1914, doctors routinely prescribed drugs to people simply to prevent withdrawals and maintain normalcy. When the act was passed, doctors were no longer allowed to engage in this practice and could only prescribe drugs for a "bonafide medical reason". Almost overnight, the illicit drug market was born (Herzberg, 2020).

The actions taken in Merseyside influenced the implementation of harm reduction programs in North America and Switzerland. The first harm reduction conference – The International Conference on the Reduction of Drug Related Harm – was held in 1990 in Liverpool, Merseyside's largest city. The International Harm Reduction Coalition was established at the conference in Warsaw in 1996. The conference has been used as a jumping off point for regions of the world interested in this innovative approach for substance use. When the conference was held in São Paulo, Brazil, in 1998, it ignited discussions about harm reduction in South America. The concept and practice of harm reduction also began getting endorsements from major health entities such as the World Health Organization, which announced their support at the 2002 conference in Slovenia (O'Hare, 2007).

Concepts

The concepts behind harm reduction were developed by the Harm Reduction Coalition (https://harmreduction.org/about-us/principles-of-harm-reduction/) and have been adopted by harm reduction focused programs and centers around the world. Below is a review of these concepts and Exercise 1 will allow you to brainstorm ways in which these concepts apply to working with adolescents.

1. Accepts that substance use is a part of society. Believes that working to reduce the harms associated with use is more beneficial than ignoring or condemning use.
   The War on Drugs established a militaristic and criminal justice approach to people who sell and use drugs. These policies supported the belief that long prison sentences and collateral sanctions such as voter disenfranchisement would discourage and even eliminate the use of illegal drugs. As a result, the US ended up as the country with the largest percentage of their population incarcerated in the world (Fair & Walmsley, 2021). The harm reduction approach moved away from punishment and towards a public health framework for substance use. People participate in potentially harmful activities every day. From sexual intercourse, to driving a car. Rather than forbid or condemn these activities due to risk, we educate people on how to make these activities safer. We discuss condom use and consent. We provide cars with seat belts and install traffic signals. These methods are more effective at reducing the harms associated with having sex or driving a car than simply outlawing these behaviors or ignoring the risks associated with them.
2. Acknowledges that substance use is complicated and multi-faceted. Recognizes that there is a spectrum of use, from abstinence to experimentation to regular use, and that there are steps that can be taken to reduce the chance of harm across the spectrum of use.

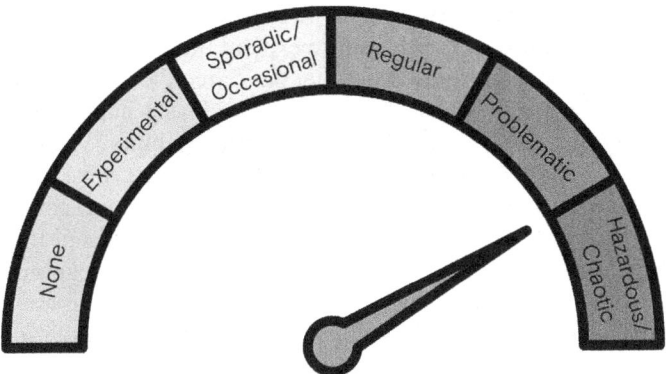

Spectrum of Substance Use

Figure 1.1 Spectrum of Substance Use.

"All use is abuse" was a common assertion during the height of the drug war. This seems a bit hypocritical given that we only apply it to illicit substances and not to legal drugs like alcohol, nicotine, or caffeine. On the one hand, someone can drink alcohol, even daily, and escape the accusations of being addicted to it. But someone who uses an illicit drug can be labeled as an "addict" simply based on use itself. Harm reduction by contrast, acknowledges that substance use, ALL substance use, exists on a spectrum.

On one side there is complete abstinence, and on the other side is chaotic, potentially hazardous use. Most people are in between the two extremes, including those who experiment, use occasionally, or even use regularly without harm. The recognition of this spectrum is even more difficult when it comes to adolescents. For minors, there is a desire to take an all or nothing approach, viewing all substance use as problematic. The trouble with this approach is that, like adults, different levels of substance use require different approaches and taking the wrong approach can actually make things worse. In addition to substance use itself being a spectrum, harm reduction scholars like Scott Kellogg posit that harm reduction interventions are a spectrum as well. In abstinence-focused treatment, the goal of the intervention is to see a complete stoppage of substance use. However, in harm reduction, the goals are also on a spectrum, referred to as gradualism. Staying alive is the primary goal, followed by maintaining health, and then getting better. In this context, harm reduction may be seen as a pathway to abstinence, by taking a course determined best by the client, and focusing on staying alive as the primary goal, rather than stopping drug use (Kellogg, 2003). In this book, we will apply this principle of harm reduction when talking about how we determine the potential harms and risks specific to where the adolescent is on the spectrum of use and what other life and social factors may be impacting the likelihood of harm, as well as having a client-centered approach to how a successful outcome is defined.

3. Focuses on quality of life as an indicator of success rather than the ability to maintain abstinence.

In many traditional mutual-aid groups like Alcoholics Anonymous and Narcotics Anonymous, success is defined by abstinence. In these programs specifically, participants are given chips celebrating the number of days they have abstained from alcohol and drugs.

(Alcoholics Anonymous, 2025) We are not here to diminish the success that some have found with this approach. Rather, we want to expand the definition of success beyond the narrow metric of abstinence and recognize that there are other indicators that may be more relevant to some. Hazardous substance use can negatively impact physical and mental health, family relationships, housing and employment stability, and other factors. When these areas of life are threatened, the urge can be to tackle the substance use first if that is believed to be the root cause. However, ensuring that housing and employment are maintained and that personal health is stabilized can create improvement in one's life separate from the sole focus on drug using behavior. The harm reduction approach uses multiple indicators of success outside of substance use as a way to work on and acknowledge the many factors that contribute to a person's overall level of health and functioning.

4. Promotes policies and programs rooted in nonjudgment that provide and encourage respect for participants and communities.
Wearing the label of "illegal drug user" attracts a high level of stigma in the United States. Beliefs about self-respect, self-control, and personal motivation are wrapped into the identity of someone who uses illicit substances. Society is taught that a person who uses illicit substances does not respect themselves, and therefore we as a society are discouraged from giving them respect as well. Harm reduction takes the approach of nonjudgment and embraces the belief that all people deserve respect, whether or not they choose to use substances. This belief extends beyond individual users and into the communities formed by people seeking mutual support and services. During the height of the HIV/AIDS epidemic, LGBTQ+ communities also faced stigma and disrespect due to inaccurate beliefs about the transmission of the disease. Faced with social disdain and isolation, community became even more important as a lifeline and source of protection. When we talk about nonjudgment and respect, we are not only talking about individuals but the communities they form in response to social discrimination.

5. Includes the voices of people who do or have used substances in the creation of policies and programs.
The act of paternalism often takes power away from those deemed to be unable to make good decisions on their own behalf. When someone is identified as an illicit substance user, the assumption is often made that they are incapable of making their own good decisions. However, research shows that people who use illicit substances do put thought into their decisions and work to make choices that will support their own health and safety (Cruz, 2015). And yet, many drug policies and programs support the idea that this population cannot be trusted to make good decisions. Adolescents who use substances are even more vulnerable to paternalism due to their choices and also their age. Harm reduction supports the idea that people who use drugs (PWUD), even young people, should have a voice when creating policies and programs that impact them, and that they can advocate on their own behalf. The San Francisco Drug Users Union (www.sfduu.org) was founded in 2007 as an organization run by people who use drugs. Their drop-in center includes syringe access, but also access to bathrooms, water, food, and medical care referrals. They also participate in advocacy efforts and partner with local public health and harm reduction agencies to expand care and empower members of their community.

6. Supports that people who use drugs (PWUD) have the power to act as agents of change and safety in their own lives and the lives of those in their communities.
Many traditional drug treatment programs involve an admission of powerlessness on the part of the person seeking treatment. However, harm reduction supports the idea that

people who use drugs, even problematically, have the power to not only make their lives safer, but to change them completely. By coming from a place of empowerment and engagement, individuals involved in harm reduction programs are encouraged to learn about how to increase their safety and how to bring that message back to the members of their communities. Research by Marlatt and Witkiewitz (2002) emphasizes the importance of including the client in defining their own needs and desired outcomes from an intervention and to acknowledge the multi-faceted aspect of behavior change not only from within, but in relation to the person-in-environment. Peer education and peer networks are a crucial part of harm reduction. This can be especially valuable for adolescents, who are more likely to listen to peers than the adults in their lives. Peer support for adolescents trying to address the impacts of substance use in their lives has shown to be a successful approach (Paquette et al., 2019) Working with teens on how to be agents of change not only for themselves but for other teens they care about is an approach that instills a sense of power and not powerlessness. This includes addressing self-efficacy, or the beliefs of the client that they are able to make a change, in addition to self-determination which supports that the client has autonomy and a choice in what happens to them and what treatment goals they create. Traditionally, in the context of substance use, this belief was focused on the ability to stay abstinent. However, harm reduction research encourages the broadening of self-efficacy goals and self-determination to include any change in substance using behavior that addresses risk reduction and is decided on by the client (Richards et al., 2021; Schwebel et al., 2024).

7. Understands the role that racism, sexism, poverty, and trauma play in both access to services and vulnerability to hazardous substance use.

   Certain groups of people are more likely to be arrested and incarcerated for illicit substance use. People of color and people without financial means are more vulnerable to drug laws due to racism and the high costs of fighting the criminal justice system. Former incarceration is associated with economic indicators such as food and housing instability (Sugie, 2015). Of Black men born in 2001, 1 in 5 is likely to be imprisoned during their lifetime (Robey et al., 2023). People of color currently represent about 7 out of 10 of those incarcerated. And, in 2022, 46% of those in federal prison were incarcerated on drug charges (Carson & Kluckow, 2023). The collateral sanctions associated with being identified as a substance user can result in more serious impacts for women who are usually the primary caregivers. Loss of child custody and the intersection of sexism can make it more difficult for women to seek help and to maintain economic stability after experiencing criminal justice involvement. Between 1980 and 1997, the number of women who were incarcerated rose by 573%, compared to a rise of 294% among men. And two-thirds of incarcerated women were mothers to children under 18, often as a single parent prior to incarceration (Mauer, Potler, & Wolf, 1999). Furthermore, trauma survivors have higher rates of problematic substance use and are more likely to experience a myriad of destabilizing factors such as mental health and employment issues. They may also be more likely to lack a strong support system. Fifty-seven percent of incarcerated women report a history of abuse and 33% report having been raped prior to incarceration (Mauer, Potler, & Wolf, 1999). Additionally, adverse childhood experiences (ACEs) are significantly predictive of hazardous substance use later in life (He et al., 2022). For this reason, harm reduction recognizes the impact of these societal and personal experiences on both vulnerability to problematic substance use and lack of access to services. Concerted efforts are made to reach out to and support people who may experience discrimination and a heightened need for services. There is also an effort to address these disparities through social justice work.

8. Recognizes that substance use can lead to very real harms both at a personal and societal level.

Finally, opponents of harm reduction often claim that this approach downplays the harms of substance use. However, this is not the case. Harm reduction absolutely recognizes the real harms that can come from substance use, whether that is dependence, overdose, or life instability. There is also a recognition of the impact of substance use on public health and safety, and family relationships. It is actually BECAUSE of this recognition of risk that harm reduction seeks to address it, rather than focusing solely on use itself. It should also again be noted that the vast majority of people who use illicit substances do so without incident (Hart, 2013). Rather than perpetuate the falsehood that all use is abuse, harm reduction recognizes the various ways in which drugs can be used and the potential harms that stem from method of ingestion, set and setting. Taking this nuanced approach does not ignore the risks, but rather allows practitioners, service providers and users themselves to take a pragmatic approach and focus on behaviors that can increase safety.

Chapter 2

Examples of Harm Reduction in the Current Substance Use Landscape

Examples of Harm Reduction in the Current Substance Use Landscape

While many people understand and support the concepts behind harm reduction, allowing programs based on these concepts has proven difficult. Partly because of the idea that punishment and condemnation work better than harm reduction when it comes to discouraging drug use, and partly related to the last concept we discussed above. There is the inaccurate assumption that by supporting drug *users*, you are supporting drug *use*. Even though the concepts of harm reduction explicitly state that there IS recognition of the harms that can result from substance use, the public, and especially politicians, not wanting to seem "soft on drugs" often refuse to support or fund programs that take a harm reduction approach.

Next, we will review some of these programs, the frameworks behind them, and the ways in which they illustrate the concepts of harm reduction.

Syringe access

One of the oldest forms of harm reduction, syringe access, formerly called needle exchange, developed as a way to prevent the spread of HIV and other diseases through the sharing of needles. Injection drug use (IDU) is not very common, but transmitting blood borne illnesses is a potential harm from this behavior. To reduce this harm, the effort was made to provide clean, sanitary needles to people who inject their drugs, and incentivizing the return of used needles to remove them from the population. This practice does not minimize the potential harms that come from the drugs themselves, such as overdose or dependence, but rather recognizes that the harm of disease is preventable by using clean needles. A 2014 meta-analysis by Aspinall et al. revealed a significant relationship between syringe access programs and a reduction in HIV transmission.

Syringe access programs are examples of harm reduction because they take a pragmatic approach to reducing the potential harms associated with injection drug use, primarily the spread of blood borne illnesses like HIV and Hepatitis B. They also serve as public health interventions by reducing the presence of used needles in community spaces. On the service side, they offer opportunities for people to interact with service providers, and even though treatment or desired abstinence is not a requirement for accessing the program, these options are made available should a participant desire them at some point in their interaction with the program. The belief that people who inject drugs (PWID) should have access to programs that help keep them safe, without demanding abstinence is rooted in the harm reduction principles of non-judgment, quality of life, and the ability of PWUD to make good decisions about risk reduction. Ideally, syringe access would be one component of a larger umbrella of care services. Research by Kidorf et al. (2011) demonstrated that access to concurrent syringe access and treatment options improved outcomes for participants. And a 2018 meta-analysis by Plat et al. found that syringe access programs were more effective when paired with the harm reduction program of opiate substitution. However, like many harm reduction focused programs, acceptance and adoption in the United States has been difficult.

Syringe access programs began in the 1980s in Amsterdam in an attempt to curb Hepatitis B infections among PWID. When HIV began to spread among this community, and it was discovered that it was a blood borne illness, syringe access programs were used to address the risks of this disease as well. The programs expanded to other Dutch cities, and then to the UK. Early research on these programs suggested that in addition to simply offering clean needles, programs needed to be client centered in order to attract participants. In the United States, the long held beliefs about PWUD, especially those who inject them, intersected with beliefs and feelings about the LGBTQ+ community and people who contracted HIV. This made it very difficult to implement syringe access programs. In 1985, a pilot program was planned by the New York City Department of Public Health, and subsequently vetoed by the police. Three years later, a pilot program that included evaluation was approved, albeit with strong opposition. And while the program did show promise in getting PWID into treatment, it was not widespread enough to have an impact on HIV transmissions, and was shut down in 1989. However during this time there were two other, privately funded programs, one in Tacoma, Washington, and one in New Haven, Connecticut, that were able to show a significant impact of syringe access programs on HIV and Hepatitis B transmissions. But even with research showing the positive impacts of these programs, a 1988 Federal Health and Human Services bill prohibited the use of federal funds for syringe access programs until they were proven safe and effective. This put access programs in limbo similarly to how medical cannabis is treated today. The federal government is the primary funder of studies designed to show the safety and efficacy of interventions such as syringe exchange, but they refused to fund research until safety and efficacy had been proved, a process that they primarily control through funding (Des Jarlais, 2017).

Without federal support, much of the research and funding for syringe access came from state and local governments, and private organizations like the American Foundation for AIDS Research (amFAR) and the Robert Wood Johnson Foundation (RWJF). As a result, the North American Syringe Exchange Network (NASEW) comprised 100 programs by 1997. The National Institute on Drug Abuse (NIDA) also began funding research on syringe access programs, greatly increasing the number of studies on its effectiveness. But even though the Department of Health and Human Services did rule that these programs were safe and effective in 1998, the continued moral opposition from Congress to such programs prevented then President Clinton from overturning the federal ban on funding (Des Jarlais, 2017).

The current re-emergence of injection transmitted HIV related to the growing opiate crisis in the US has reinvigorated the discussion around syringe access programs. However, even as states and localities struggle to address this issue, the continued federal ban on funding inhibits the development and expansion of these programs (Des Jarlais, 2017).

Opponents of syringe access claim that making clean needles available is enabling substance users to continue to use drugs rather than quit, and the issue itself has become highly politicized. This struggle is represented in the research. A 2017 meta-analysis on the effectiveness of syringe access programs in reducing needle sharing behavior by Sawangjit et al. found that syringe access programs were associated with lower rates of needle sharing behaviors, but that 64% of the studies they reviewed were subject to high levels of bias.

One concern over syringe access programs is that, while they provide clean needles to PWID, they do not include a safe space to use drugs. This does not address public injecting, and limits the exposure of participants to the ancillary services that have been found to enhance outcomes. Additionally, because participants must still use their substances away from the program area, addressing overdose becomes difficult. Overdose prevention facilities aim to provide clean equipment to PWUD, while also providing a safe consumption space and more readily available ancillary services.

Overdose prevention facilities

Previously called "safe injection facilities" the goal of overdose prevention facilities (OPF) is to provide a safe space for the use of drugs, one equipped with overdose treatment medications and medical professionals. Forcing people who use drugs to do so alone, or in spaces without access to Narcan or medical help increases the chance of death should an overdose occur. Like syringe access programs, OPFs do not ignore the potential risks of using illicit substances, but recognize that there are ways to reduce these risks by ensuring that consumers have safe spaces and access to emergency care. And while these programs have traditionally focused on injection drug use, there is also support for allowing other types of substance use with the same types of harm reduction and medical services. Additionally, OPFs provide access to treatment services if desired, and many also help with housing, food and employment services. Like syringe access programs, OPFs are true to the harm reduction principles around reducing risks and potential harms from substance use without demanding abstinence, a position of nonjudgment, and the belief that PWUD can make healthy decisions about how to reduce risk and the role that substances play in their lives, even while actively using.

Although Safe Consumption Sites, or Safe Injection Facilities, or Overdose Prevention Facilities are largely considered to be a modern phenomenon, the concept of providing safe spaces and clean tools to use substances dates back to the early 1900s in the United States (Jones, 2021). As previously mentioned, the 1914 Harrison Narcotics Act put an end to doctors prescribing drugs like morphine just to quell withdrawal symptoms. However, a loophole in the law concerning medical therapy allowed for the establishment of "morphine maintenance clinics", which afforded users access to medical opiates as well as a place to safely use them (Herzberg, 2020). The first of such clinics opened in Jacksonville, Florida, in 1912, and dozens were in operation in the early 1920s when they were all shut down by federal authorities (Musto, 1999).

Modern day facilities began in Bern, Switzerland, in 1986. And although there are now hundreds of such facilities across Europe, Australia, and Canada, they are not located in countries with a high prevalence of HIV transmission related to injection drug use (Beletsky et al., 2018). As with syringe access programs, the United States has struggled to open a sanctioned OPF. San Francisco worked on opening such a site for years, but was not successful other than non-sanctioned pop up facilities run by local nonprofits. Similar unsanctioned sites have opened in cities in the U.S., but often must stay hidden, making it difficult for the population they are intended for to find them. However, research on even unsanctioned facilities shows that, although overdoses do occur, their occurrence at an OPF allows for medical intervention to be administered. In one study of an unsanctioned OPF in the US, between the years of 2014 and 2019, there were 10,517 injections and 33 overdoses, none of which resulted in death (Kral et al., 2020). Safehouse, a proposed OPF in Philadelphia fell victim to a provision in the federal "Crackhouse Statute". The statute, part of the Controlled Substances Act, makes it illegal for anyone to maintain a space for the purposes of selling or using federally illegal substances. Safehouse sued the federal government for the right to open in 2019 on the grounds of the first amendment and religious freedom, but their case was dismissed in 2024 (Feldman, 2020; Leonard, 2024). In 2022, the first sanctioned US OPF opened in New York, run by an organization called OnPointNYC (Peltz, 2022).

But while the US is slowly coming to terms with the benefits of OPFs, Canada began opening unsanctioned facilities in the mid-1990s, with the first sanctioned center, Insite, opening in 2003. One misconception about OPFs is that they do not support abstinence. This is not true. Insite, located in Vancouver, is one of the only OPFs in the world that provides wrap-around services in addition to a safe place to use drugs. Visitors can choose to enter treatment or stay at their facilities to power through withdrawals. Those who work at the facility report that sometimes people come to use their services for months, or even years, until one day they say they are ready to stop using, and when that day happens, Insite is there for them (Doberstein, 2022). But, even though Canada was more open to OPFs as an intervention to reduce overdose and the transmission of HIV, it was the community of PWUD themselves who stood on the front lines to protect the centers and ensure that they stay open. This directly speaks to the harm reduction value of including the substance using community in decisions and program development that impacts them (Kerr et al., 2017).

In recent years, several US cities plus the states of New Hampshire and Vermont have approved the establishment of OPFs. In Vermont, the centers extend beyond injection drug use and include the smoking of substances like cocaine (Vermont Department of Health, 2024). This is one reason the nomenclature has shifted from "safe injection facilities" to "overdose prevention facilities". Another reason is that the main goal of these centers is not to allow drug use, but to prevent overdose. In their first three months in operation, the OPFs run by OnPointNYC stopped over 150 overdoses among their 9,500 clinic visits (Peltz, 2022).

Like syringe access programs, opponents of OPFs claim that these programs downplay the risks of substance use and take a permissive stance. However, it is quite the contrary. It is BECAUSE of the recognition of the potential harms of using these substances that OPFs exist. And research supports their success. A 2014 meta-analysis by Potier et al. found that safe injection facilities were associated with attracting marginalized PWID, safer injection conditions, access to primary care, and reducing overdose frequency and the presence of public injection drug use and discarded syringes. Additionally, they found that they were not associated with increases in drug trafficking or crime in the neighborhoods in which they were located. A 2022 systematic review conducted by Levengood et al. primarily focused on studies from Insite, found evidence of reductions in opiate related morbidity and mortality, improvements in injection behaviors and the reduction of harm, improved access to addiction treatment programs, and no increase in crime or public nuisance.

Again, beliefs about PWUD and the function of OPFs as permissive facilities versus harm reduction interventions have stood in the way of such centers opening, despite the strong research that shows their benefits to the health and wellness of this population. And while strong advocates from the arenas of public health and social welfare exist, in many cases, it has been up to the substance-using community themselves to advocate on their own behalf for centers and services that prioritize safety rather than abstinence-only approaches.

The need to organize these communities and better self-advocate has led to the emergence of another harm reduction-focused entity: drug user's unions.

Drug user's unions

One of the tenets of harm reduction is the involvement of PWUD in the formation of policies around drug use, as well as the recognition that these groups can be successful educators and peer supporters for their communities. Historically, people who choose to use substances have been viewed as irresponsible and unable to make rational choices in their own best interests. However, research suggests that this is not true, and that people, even when dealing with physical and psychological addiction, can make choices that support their own health and well-being and that of their community (Arnaud, 2021). Drug users unions were formed to support PWUD in advocating not only for policies that treat their communities fairly and humanely, but to push back against the narrative that they are incapable of actively participating in discussions about their rights and lives.

The first drug user's union, "Junkie-Bond", was established in 1977 in Rotterdam, Netherlands, and established the Medical-Social Service for Heroin Users. The main goals of the program were to gain social acceptance of drugs and drug users, decriminalize the use of drugs, and the de-psychiatric and de-medication of the drug user (van Dam, 2008). Then, in the early 1990s, the Vancouver Area Network of Drug Users (VANDU) was formed to advocate for changes in city policies around drug use in response to the HIV epidemic. It was this advocacy that led to the opening of the first safe consumption center in North America. Canada has continued to lead the way for drug user's unions with groups like the Toronto Drug User's Union, the Toronto Overdose Prevention Society, the BC-Yukon Association for Drug War Survivors, and the Canadian Association for People Who Use Drugs. These groups have been instrumental in making Canada one of the most harm reduction focused countries in the world when it comes to substance use (International Drug Policy Consortium, 2020).

Outside of North America, groups in Germany and the Netherlands have been successful at advocating for safe consumption centers and heroin prescription programs. In South Africa, the South African Network of People Who Use Drugs has been successful in advocating for harm reduction-based policies. Similar groups are located around the world in India, Russia, Australia, the UK, Georgia, Ukraine, Asia, New Zealand, Mexico, Tanzania, and Afghanistan. In the United States, which is a major center of the Drug War, drug user's unions in New York and San Francisco have worked tirelessly to shift drug policies from punishment to harm reduction. Many of the groups in these countries are part of the International Network of People Who Use Drugs (INPUD) (International Drug Policy Consortium, 2020).

In addition to advocacy, there is a role of drug user's unions in the development of research on drug use. For the academic community, the cultural competence needed to properly and effectively work with marginalized groups has been a barrier to meaningful studies. For drug user's unions, expressing their experiences and expertise in a way that is impactful in an academic setting can be difficult. Even in the context of community-based participatory research (CBPR), the power differential between the researchers and the drug user's unions complicates the process. The Urban Survivor's Union, the national drug user's union in the US, suggests that a better approach to CBPR is community driven research (CDR). CDR is different from CBPR because the research focus, methodology and process is led by the community, rather than by the academics, with the community only invited to participate in the process alongside them (Simon et al., 2021).

Safer supply/drug checking

Prohibition prevents discussions about how to make drug use safer, as the only objective is to prevent use entirely. Research supports that services like drug checking and access to safer drug supplies can greatly reduce deaths related to tainted products (Gulini et al., 2022). We saw a similar phenomenon during alcohol prohibition. During prohibition, deaths due to an unsafe supply of alcohol were common. These instances were reduced once prohibition was over and the supply was tested and regulated (Thorton, 1991). Unfortunately, drug prohibition has reduced the opportunities for these services. The RAVE Act passed in 2003 prohibited drug checking at festivals and other mass events because the presence of such services implicated the organizers as knowing that drugs were being sold and consumed at their events (U.S. Congress, 2021).

One organization, Dance Safe, founded in 1998, has been fighting against these restrictions by educating party goers on the safer use of substances and working to provide drug testing kits and medical services for people having difficult experiences. The mission of Dance Safe is: "To promote health, safety, and fulfilling experiences for people who use drugs and their communities." Dance Safe sells drug checking kits and strips through their website and provides drug education at festivals and other events. They also run the only available drug checking lab in the United States. Founded in 1999, it was handed over to the organization, Erowid, in 2001 as the Ecstasy Data Project. This was renamed Drugs Data in 2019 due to the wide range of substances that were being sent in for testing. Drugs submitted, as well as their results, are posted on the Drugs Data website (drugsdata.org) (DanceSafe, 2025). However, in April of 2024, the lab was forced to stop accepting samples when the Drug Enforcement Administration (DEA) ordered them to shut down pending administrative review (Erowid, 2025).

While most of the earlier drug checking focused on designer drugs like MDMA, the emergence of Fentanyl in the drug supply has reignited the discussion about drug checking and its role in reducing deaths. In December 2024, the DEA reported that, for the first time since 2018, drug overdose deaths decreased in the United States, down 14.5% between June 2023 and June 2024. However, 70% of the drug overdose deaths were due to opioids such as Fentanyl. The DEA's testing laboratory reports that five out of 10 pills tested contained a lethal dose of Fentanyl (DEA, 2024). The rise of Fentanyl overdoses has pushed the Federal Government to finally accept and promote drug checking as a harm reduction strategy, at least in this one narrow circumstance. The Centers for Disease Control has a web page dedicated to promoting the use of Fentanyl testing strips (CDC, 2025). However, it should be noted that the CDC website now bears a disclaimer saying that it is in the process of being modified to comply with President Trump's Executive Orders, so it is unclear if such information will be provided in the future. As of the writing of this book, Fentanyl Test Strips are available for purchase on Amazon.com. However, other illicit substances are also at risk of contamination and safer supply laws should be more universal rather than only being used for certain drugs. Opinions about the people who use certain drugs may impact whether there is support for safer supply. The use of designer drugs by middle class teens and young adults makes drug checking more palatable because it is being done in the context of saving youth lives. Once the opioid crisis began impacting the White middle class, calls for safer supply and drug checking amplified. However, users of drugs like methamphetamine and other stimulants still receive high levels of stigma creating barriers for safer supply programs. Regulated and prescribed stimulants could act as substitutes for cocaine and other drugs currently being obtained from an unregulated market and therefore at risk for contamination (Fleming et al., 2020).

Chapter 3

Drug Using Behavior in Adolescence

Drug Using Behavior in Adolescence

Part of the current model of "Just Say No", fear-based drug prevention programs for adolescents is based on the premise that adolescent substance use is a problem pervasive enough to warrant a highly paternalistic approach. From the very early drug propaganda films of the 1960s and 1970s, parents have been fed a steady stream of "truths" regarding how adolescent substance use works. It usually goes something like, a teen from a good home with loving supportive parents falls in with a "bad crowd" and, in a moment of weakness, is pressured into trying marijuana. This "gateway" inevitably leads down a path of criminality and life failure with harder drugs like heroin leading the way. In fact, in many of these films, teens are shown trying a joint and then, in the very next frame, injecting with a needle.

This imagery was a powerful motivator for parents to do whatever it took, even putting their teen in jail, to save them from a life of addiction, and maybe even more importantly, failure. It was every middle-class suburban parent's nightmare that their child would amount to nothing, and drug use was a convenient scapegoat that played upon that fear.

But what does the data say about substance use in adolescence? If the gateway theory held true, we would see similar rates of the use of all drugs. If the removal of criminal penalties also removed deterrents for use, we would see adolescent use of now legal substances like cannabis rise in states where there is now a regulated market. But this is not the picture painted by national government administered surveys like the National Survey on Drug Use and Health (NSDUH) or the Monitoring the Future (MTF) survey. Let's dive into what the data do say about the prevalence and trends in adolescent substance use.

Trends in adolescent substance use

Analyzing data from the 1970–2020 Monitoring the Future (MTF) study, Johnston and colleagues provide a trend analysis of adolescent substance use, access, and perceptions (Miech et al., 2025).

The MTF study only surveyed 12th graders until 1990, when they began surveying 8th and 10th graders as well. For 12th graders, lifetime use of any illicit substance rose from the mid-1970s to the early 1980s and then began to decline. This decline continued until the early 1990s. At this point, 8th and 10th graders were included in the survey. Through the 1990s, lifetime use of any illicit substance rose for all grades and topped out in 1997. It has been on a steady decline ever since. A similar pattern was observed for past 12-month use of any illicit substance, although overall rates of this behavior are lower. There is a similar pattern when looking at lifetime and past 12-month use of any illicit substance except for cannabis.

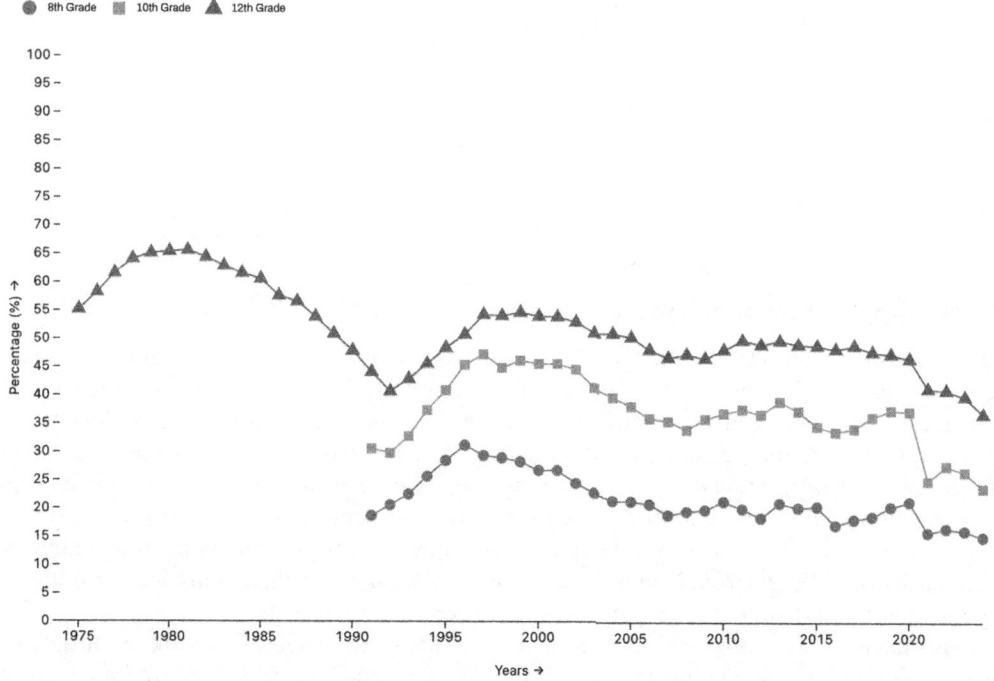

Figure 3.1 Monitoring the Future, Institute for Social Research, University of Michigan.

Again, although the pattern is the same, the fact that cannabis is the most widely used illicit substance among teens flattens the overall rates when cannabis is removed from the equation.

When looking just at cannabis, we see a similar pattern, with past 12-month use rates increasing slightly in the late 1970s, before falling sharply in the 1980s and into the early 1990s, when they began to creep up again. This increase was observed until 1996 when rates again began to fall. All grades exhibited a decline in reported use from 1996 until around 2008 when use rates flattened out. Of note, the move to legalize cannabis for recreational use beginning in 2012 did not seem to impact use rates among adolescents. Regarding perceived risk, the percentage of students who saw "great risk" in regular cannabis use was inversely related to use rates. As use rates rise, perceived risk falls and as rates fall, perceive risk rises. However, although use rates have remained fairly stable since 2008, perceived risk has continued to decline. This suggests that legalization may impact perceived risk even if it does not impact the decision to consume. The disapproval of regular cannabis use rose during the 1980s and remained stable until it began declining around 2004. Perceived availability of cannabis was added to MTF in 1990. The percent of teens reporting that cannabis was easy to obtain rose throughout the 1990s in line with consumption rates, topping out in 1998. It then began to decline. It should be noted that perceived availability continued to decline as use rates flattened out. Prior to legalization use rates increased as perceived access increased. Post legalization, perceived access dropped while use rates remained flat.

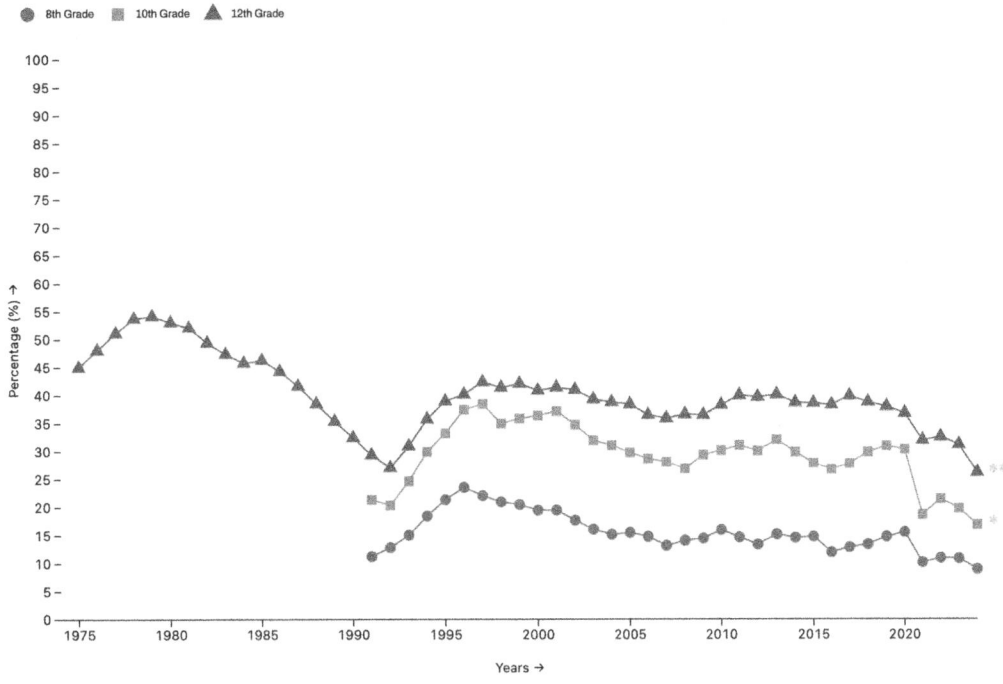

Figure 3.2 Monitoring the Future, Institute for Social Research, University of Michigan.

Current landscape according to the data

To better understand the current rates of substance use among adolescents as well as recent trends, we turn to two of the longest running surveys administered by the US Government. While not perfect in their methodology, these surveys have been conducted for five decades in all 50 states and provide a good source of information when it comes to trends as well as current prevalence. However, it should also be noted that measuring adolescent substance use (or the use of illicit substances among any population) can be difficult. Some teens feel the need to hide their use due to legality, stigma or pressures from home (even though the survey is anonymous) and others feel the need to make false claims about their use to appear tough or more experienced than they are. The truth is, as long as substance use is tied to morality and personality, rather than being simply a health behavior, people will hide or exaggerate the truth based on who they want to appear to be. With that being said, let's take a look at the data. To assess current use of illicit and legal drugs by adolescents, we looked at two data sources, Monitoring the Future (MTF) and the National Survey on Drug Use and Health (NSDUH). MTF is funded by NIDA and has been administered by the University of Michigan's Institute for Social Research since 1975. MTF collects data on substance use trends and attitudes among adolescents (8th, 10th, and 12th graders) and adults. The NSDUH is funded by Substance Abuse and Mental Health Services Administration (SAMHSA) and collects data on substance use, mental health, and treatment trends among adolescents

20 Harm Reduction Approaches with Adolescents Who Use Substances

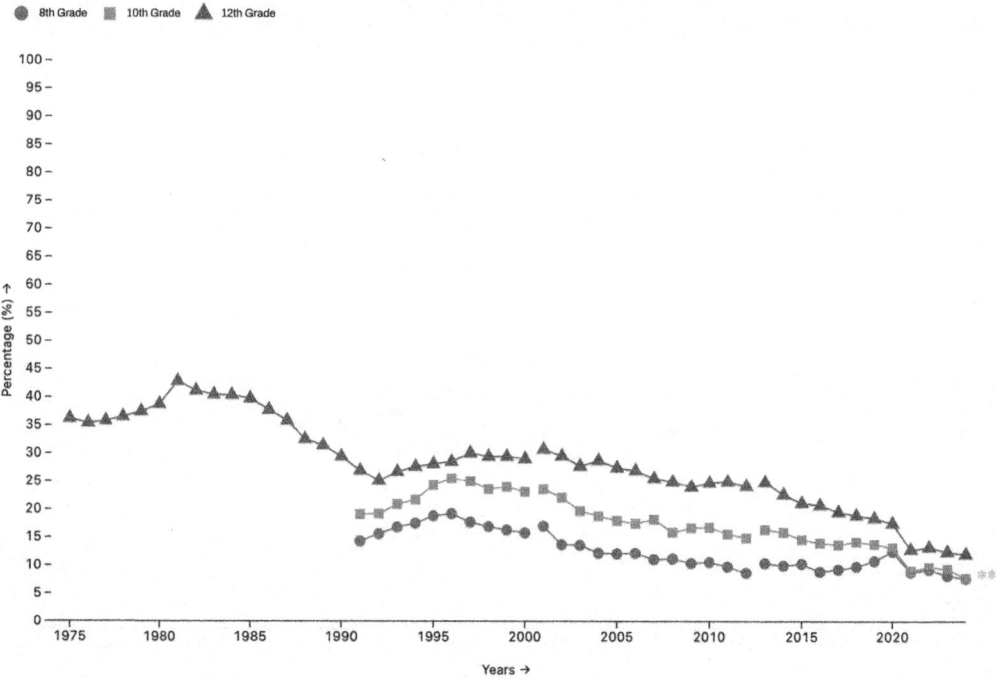

Figure 3.3 Monitoring the Future, Institute for Social Research, University of Michigan.

and adults. For the purposes of this book, we will focus on the data concerning school-age adolescents.

Prevalence of drug and alcohol use among adolescents

First, let's look at the most recent data from Monitoring the Future (2023). Table 3.1 shows the percentage of students in each grade level reporting 30-day past use of various illicit and legal substances. We chose to report the past 30-day data rather than past year or lifetime because the purpose of this book is to present strategies for working with adolescents who are currently using substances. We will refer to the difference between lifetime and 30-day past use data when discussing experimental versus regular use.

Overall, past 30-day use of illicit substances is low among all age groups. Even though MTF categorizes marijuana as an illicit substance for the purposes of this survey, 36 states have some form of cannabis access, whether it be only for medical purposes or for adult use and medical purposes, so many of these students live in a market where cannabis is not an illicit substance. Cannabis accounts for most of the illicit drug use across grades, with nearly 20% of 12th graders reporting past 30-day use. The rates of alcohol use among this age group are higher at 24%. The rates of alcohol use are higher among all grades when compared to cannabis. Other than cannabis, inhalants are the most commonly used illicit substance among 8th graders, which could reflect a lack of access to other substances while inhalants can be

Drug Using Behavior in Adolescence   21

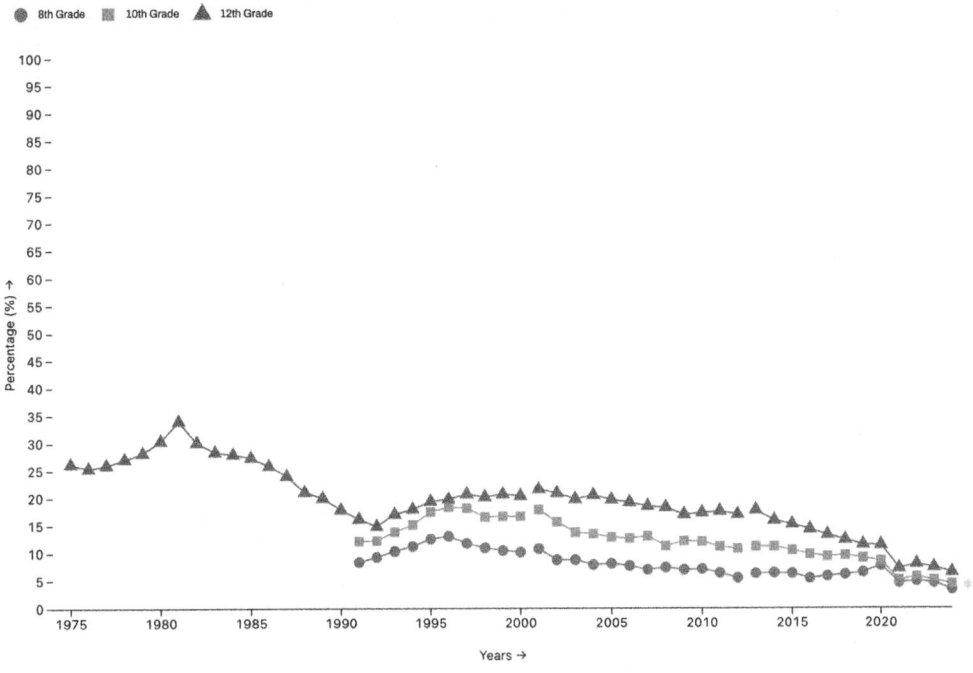

Figure 3.4 Monitoring the Future, Institute for Social Research, University of Michigan.

Table 3.1 Percent of 8th, 10th, and 12th graders reporting past 30 day substance use (Monitoring the Future Survey, 2023)

	Any illicit drug	Any illicit drug other than marijuana	Marijuana	Inhalants	Hallucinogens	LSD	Hallucinogens other than LSD	Ecstasy (MDMA)
8th	6.5%	2.6%	4.7%	2.6%	.5%	.3%	.2%	.3%
10th	11.3%	2.3%	10.3%	.9%	.8%	.4%	.7%	.3%
12th	19.8%	3.4%	18.4%	1.2%	1.6%	.4%	1.5%	.3%

easily obtained. 10th graders are more likely to use amphetamines than other illicit substances, which could reflect using Adderall without a prescription. And 12th graders use hallucinogens that are not LSD (likely psilocybin mushrooms) more frequently than they use other illicit substances.

In Table 3.2, looking at substances that are federally legal, even if they are age-restricted, while 5.9%, 13.7%, and 24.3% of 8th, 10th, and 12th graders, respectively, say they have used alcohol in the past 30 days, less than half of those groups report being "drunk". This speaks both to the fact that people can consume alcohol without reaching a level of severe intoxication, but also that, unlike the other substances listed, there is a recognition that drinking

Table 3.2 Past 30-day use of alcohol, cigarettes and vaping among 8th, 10th, and 12th graders (Monitoring the Future Survey, 2023)

	Cocaine	Crack	Heroin	Amphetamine	Tranquilizers
8th	.3%	.2%	.3%	1.6%	.4%
10th	.4%	.2%	.2%	1.3%	.4%
12th	.4%	.3%	.1%	1.1%	.3%

alcohol does not automatically render someone drunk. The "all use is abuse" claim made with illicit substances is not being applied to alcohol because alcohol is legal. We will revisit this issue when we review the NSDUH data on treatment admissions among adolescents. Harm reduction encourages the recognition that, even among adolescents, there are variances in substance consumption that contribute to their risks and potential harms.

Harm reduction also views vaping as a safer way to consume nicotine or cannabis than smoking it. This is a tricky subject to navigate with adolescents, because even though vaping may be less harmful to their health, the stealth nature of vaping may make it easier for adolescents to engage in that behavior than smoking. We have seen, over the past decade, a transition among teens from smoking to vaping nicotine as evidenced by the MTF data. According to the MTF data, while less than 3% of students in each of the grades report smoking cigarettes in the past 30 days, 7%, 12%, and 17%, respectively, report vaping nicotine. The rates of vaping marijuana account for most of the marijuana use reported by the three grade levels, showing that it is the preferred method of ingestion for adolescents. The question is, would they still consume marijuana as often if vaping did not exist? Many would argue they would not, since there are reports of marijuana vaping in schools and other places where smoking would be too apparent (Wang et al., 2024).

In addition to the vaping of cannabis, vaping tobacco in the form of e-cigarettes is becoming more common among adolescents. Findings from the 2024 National Youth Tobacco Survey and reported by the FDA, show that 7.8% of high school and 3.5% of middle school students currently use e-cigarettes. Twenty-six percent of users say they use e-cigarettes daily, and 38% have used them at least 20 of the last 30 days. Eighty-eight percent report using flavored e-cigarettes, and over half reported using a disposable device versus a refillable one (FDA, 2025).

While many adults use e-cigarettes as a form of harm reduction to cut down on smoking, teens may be using them for different reasons but still in the context of harm reduction. An analysis of the 2015 and 2016 Monitoring the Future Survey by Evans-Polce et al., revealed that 63% of 12th graders who vape say they were doing it for taste and entertainment, while only 7% said they were doing it to replace cigarettes. Additional analyses of the 2015 Monitoring the Future Study, which included teens from 8th, 10th, and 12th grades, found similar results, with experimentation (53%), taste (37%) and boredom (24%) listed as the top reasons for vaping. As with the previous study, substitution for cigarettes was uncommon (Patrick et al., 2016).

From a harm reduction perspective, it should be noted that reasons for vaping differ among those who use daily and those who use occasionally. A 2024 study by Patrick et al., analyzing data from the 2021 and 2023 Monitoring the Future Surveys, revealed that among 12th graders reporting near daily vaping, 70% said they used to relax or relieve tension. Among those across grades who reported vaping in the past 30 days, 56% reported using to relax or relieve tension.

This dropped to 49% among those who reported any vaping in the past 12 months. However, infrequent vapers were more likely to report using to have a good time with friends, 30% versus 21% for near daily users. Finally, near daily users were more likely to report using vapes instead of cigarettes (33%) versus past 30 day (17%) and past 12 month (14%) users. This suggests that regular vaping is more likely to be related to addressing anxiety and smoking substitution, and less related to the social experience. Also of note, regular vapers were more likely to admit being dependent on vaping (43%) versus those who have used in the past 30 days (17%) or past 12 months (13%). This data suggests implications for how vaping is approached with teens based on their frequency of and motivations for use.

Prevalence of experimental versus regular or problematic use

To explore the patterns of consumption we are going to look at the prevalence of adolescents who used a substance 10 times or more in their lifetime but have not used it in the past year. MTF only reports this data for 12th graders, and when N=50+ who have used the substance more than 10 times. Because of this, substances with a very low use rate are not represented.

As seen in Table 3.3, data show that, across substances, there is a percentage of 12th graders who engaged in abstention even after using that substance 10+ times. This shows that substance use is episodic, and not automatically an escalating behavior. When looking at lifetime, past year, and past 30 day use, across grades, the percentage of youth engaging in the behavior declines as frequency increases. For example, for 8th graders and marijuana, 5.2% report using one to two times in their lifetime and .6% report using 40+ times in the past 30 days. This pattern repeats across ages and substances, showing that there is a difference between occasional and regular use, and that most of the use reported by adolescents is occasional. We will revisit this when we talk about strategies for working with adolescents as regular and occasional use warrant different approaches. Working with an adolescent who has used cannabis one to two times in their lifetime looks different than working with one who has used 40+ times in the past month.

Prevalence of substance use disorder and treatment

Now we will review data from the NSDUH to examine the prevalence of Substance Use Disorder and Alcohol Abuse/Dependence and treatment among adolescents aged 12–17. It should be noted that, when it comes to adolescent use of illicit substances, all use is typically viewed as abuse. Teens caught with cannabis may be diagnosed with Cannabis Use Disorder (which was added to the DSM in 2013) from any level of use, regardless of its regularity or intensity, especially if use was occurring at school, or viewed as disruptive to other social and

Table 3.3 12th graders who report abstaining for at least one year after using a substance more than 10 times (Monitoring the Future Survey, 2023)

	Alcohol	Been Drunk	Flavored alcoholic beverage	Cigarettes	Any vaping	Vaping Nicotine	Vaping Marijuana
8th	5.9%	1.5%	3.2%	1.1%	8.7%	7%	4.2%
10th	13.7%	5.1%	7.9%	2.3%	14.4%	11.9%	8.5%
12th	24.3%	12.5%	17.9%	2.9%	22.1%	16.9%	13.7%

Table 3.4 12th graders who report abstaining for at least one year after using a substance more than 10 times (Monitoring the Future Survey, 2023)

	Marijuana	Hallucinogens	Amphetamines	Alcohol	Been Drunk	Cigarettes
12th	4.9%	6.3%	27.8%	1.5%	4.2%	56.1%

Table 3.5 Substance use disorder past year ages 12-17 (National Survey on Drug Use and Health, 2023)

	Opioids	Cocaine	Prescription Drugs	Heroin	Amphetamine	Tranquilizers or Sedatives
12-17	1.2%	.2%	2.3%	<.1%	.1%	.5%

Table 3.6 Past year treatment for alcohol and drug use among those 12–17 (National Survey on Drug Use and Health, 2023)

	Alcohol	Any illicit drug	Both alcohol and drugs
12-17	.8%	2.4%	.3%

academic activities. This is not always the case with alcohol, where underaged use may result in removal from extracurricular activities, or if caught drinking at home, punishment from parents, but will likely not result in a diagnosis of alcohol abuse or dependence on these grounds alone. As can be seen from the data in Tables 3.4 and 3.5, the rates of dependence on illicit substances other than cannabis are very low because their overall rates of use are very low.

Related to the "all use is abuse" narrative, the rates of Cannabis Use Disorder are higher than Alcohol Use Disorder, even though, as shown in Table 3.1, past 30-day alcohol use is higher for all grades than cannabis use. Interestingly, the NSDUH does not classify alcohol as an illicit substance and therefore does not ask about use, even though alcohol is illicit for this age group. The rates of diagnosed dependence/abuse involving prescription drugs are almost as high as alcohol and the rate of opioid dependence is higher than that of heroin, suggesting that teens are accessing alternative forms of opioids, most likely as Oxycontin (opioids are not included in the prescription drug category).

Again, as seen in Table 3.6, although rates of alcohol are higher than rates of illicit substance use, treatment for drugs remains higher than that for alcohol. This is not a commentary on the relative safety of alcohol versus drug use for adolescents, but more an observation about how the social acceptance and legality of a substance can impact the flexibility of what is experimentation and what is abuse. That being said, there are risks for adolescents who use alcohol and drugs. In the next section we will review the research on the progression of drug use during adolescents and the risks associated with age of onset, environmental conditions and underlying mental and physical health issues. By identifying the differential population-based risks associated with use, we can better tailor harm reduction strategies that are person-focused and client-centered. We can also better consider factors beyond substance use that might serve as risk or protective factors.

Chapter 4

Substance Use in Adolescence
Potential Harms and Suggested Approaches

Substance Use In Adolescence: Potential Harms and Suggested Approaches

Because this is a textbook focused on harm reduction, it is important to examine what the potential harms are, so that strategies for reduction can be created and implemented. And while we know that cannabis poses risks of a different nature than the use of some other drugs (including prescription drugs and alcohol), these risks do have the potential to lead to harms, even if those harms are not fatal. One of the risks most commonly cited for cannabis use by adolescents is referred to as the Gateway Theory. This assumption, represented in anti-drug films from the 1960s and '70s and continued throughout the D.A.R.E. era of the 1980s and '90s, suggests that the simple act of using cannabis will cause a teen to try more dangerous substances like heroin. Many of these early anti-drug films showed teenagers being goaded into trying a cannabis joint, and then moving swiftly into injection drug use. The message for parents was clear: you may think cannabis is harmless, but if your teen uses it, they will be moved to try other drugs that are very harmful. Stopping cannabis use stops the progression into other drug use. But is there any truth to the Gateway Theory, and are there risks of using other drugs for those who try cannabis as teens? The answer is not simple and has to do with more than just cannabis use (Kleinig, 2015).

Denise Kandel is one of the foremost experts in the Gateway Theory and has taken it apart to see what might drive the progression of substance use. In her study of a cohort of 1,160 adults who were followed from grades 10–11 to ages 34–35, she looked at substance use and the conditions in which progression occurred. She included substances like tobacco and alcohol in her analysis as well as illicit substances. Kandel discovered that, rather than cannabis being the initial entry into substance use, it was more likely to be alcohol or tobacco. And while there was a high rate of use of other illicit substances among those who used cannabis, the highest rates of cannabis use and other illicit substances were among those who used alcohol. Kandel posits that while consumption of licit substances like tobacco and alcohol often precede the use of illicit substances like cannabis, they are not stepping stones. Using one does not cause the use of another, and many people stop at certain stages of use and do not progress. Relevant for this book is the finding that earlier onset and frequency of use can predict a higher likelihood of problematic use later on. It is suggested that early intervention can address this. Kandel also concludes that there are other factors related to early onset of use that might support the progression of use, other than the drug itself (Kandel, Yamaguchi, & Chen, 1992).

Additional research on the Gateway Theory has found that polysubstance initiation and the presence of mental health risks intensify the likelihood of drug use progression and intensity (Attaiaa et al., 2016; Secades-Villa et al., 2014). This suggests that, when discussing harm reduction for substance use among adolescents, it is important to consider age of onset, polysubstance use, and mental health risk factors. But also that alcohol and tobacco should not be discounted in the equation simply because they are legally regulated for adults.

How should therapists and other mental health professionals approach the desire to use harm reduction for an issue as contentious and morally laden as adolescent substance use? While most discussions of teen substance use take on an emotional and paternalistic tone, harm reduction is completely pragmatic. It is understandable why parents react to teen substance use in a protective and anxious manner, as we will discuss in the upcoming sections, there are real dangers to hazardous substance use in the teen years related to physical, psychological, and social functioning. And, these harms are connected to the age of onset, environment, and other risk taking behaviors. However, the goal of harm reduction is not to proselytize about the dangers of drugs, but rather to provide actionable steps to reduce potential risks. As a mental health professional, delivering education on these strategies from a place of nonjudgment is at the core of harm reduction as an intervention (Collins & Clifaseri, 2023). Another key component for a harm reduction therapist, and something that is especially difficult to implement when working with younger people, is the notion that the client is the expert in their own life. So many therapeutic modalities rely on the professional being the expert, which creates the paternalistic approach commonly a part of even evidence-informed treatment methods. In harm reduction, the client informs the therapist of their goals and desired outcomes. In social work we like to say, a client has the right to make their own decisions, even if we, as social workers, disagree with that decision. The innate desire to protect teens from harm may make it difficult to allow them to lead the goals of their intervention, and of course, efforts to disrupt behaviors that are truly risky should be made. But client autonomy and participation in defining the goals of the therapeutic process is one thing that differentiates harm reduction from interventions more typically found in traditional approaches to substance abuse treatment. Finally, as a clinician, it is important to acknowledge your own privilege and power (Collins & Clifaseri, 2023). The dynamic in adolescent therapy is more heavy handed towards the therapist than when both participants are adults. This dynamic may make it more uncomfortable for the adolescent to open up about the true nature of their substance use and its contributing factors. It may also make the identification of desired outcomes a rockier road as the adolescent may believe they have to say certain things in order to "please" the therapist and/or their parents. The concept of harm reduction becomes an important part of the therapist/client relationship and understanding its nature is likely necessary for the teen to open up and talk honestly about their current behavior, and what they want the outcome of the intervention to be. They may believe that complete abstinence is the only thing the therapist wants to hear. They may say this in order to "do the right thing" while continuing to use substances. This creates a missed opportunity for a discussion about safer using behaviors.

Potential harms and outcomes for adolescents who engage in early drug and alcohol use

While harm reduction does not focus just on substance use as a potential source of harm in an adolescent's life, it also does not downplay the very real risks and harms that can come from the early use of alcohol and drugs. Substance use in adolescence, as well as other life and environmental circumstances can predict substance use as an adult (Merlin et al., 2004). In addition to environmental vulnerabilities, teens have developmental and social vulnerabilities that can negatively interact with the use of intoxicating substances. At the same time, we have stressed the importance of not treating all use as abuse. The approach taken to adolescent substance use should be related to not only the use pattern, but the umbrella of other behaviors and circumstances as well as the substance in question. While all substances may present some level of risk, the potential for serious harm such as fatal overdose, varies.

Adolescent specific presentation of symptoms

The ways in which adolescents present with the symptoms of problematic substance use may be different from the chronic use symptoms exhibited by adults. Additionally, the ways in which problematic substance use may show up in an adolescent's life is unique because their roles and responsibilities are unique to this stage of life. From a harm reduction perspective, focus should be on the ways in which substance use is bringing risks and potential harm into their lives and on strategies to reduce these risks and chance of harm, regardless of what that looks like for the substance use itself. If a teen is drinking on the weekends and then driving home intoxicated, then the more immediate focus may be on eliminating the risk of driving while intoxicated, and then focusing on the weekend drinking behavior. If the weekend drinking behavior includes intoxication to the point of alcohol poisoning, then that might become a dual priority with the cessation of drinking and driving. Binge drinking has been associated with other risky health related behaviors, as well as increased difficulty transitioning into young adulthood. From a risk reduction perspective, addressing binge drinking specifically rather than all alcohol use as an umbrella behavior could have a greater impact on the reduction of hazardous behaviors (Marlatt & Witkiewitz, 2002). If a teen is using cannabis once or twice a month and also in danger of flunking their classes, the school issue may take precedence as failing out may cause more harm than occasional cannabis use. This approach is easier said than done for a couple of reasons. First, parents do not want their teen engaged in ANY activity that may be harmful, so choosing to prioritize rather than take on everything at once may feel counterintuitive. Secondly, we are taught that substance use, especially for teens, is the most harmful thing they can engage in, no matter how frequently it is happening. Turning focus away from non-problematic substance use and towards something that is presenting higher risk is difficult for many parents. The complexity of adolescent substance use and its approaches is why understanding the symptoms and differences between experimentation and problematic use are essential. For example, research by Stockwell et al. (2004) found that younger teens who use substances are more likely to be at higher risk than older teens.

As we have discussed, for adolescents, problematic substance use is often related to physical, psychological, or social distress. While experimenting with substances like alcohol and cannabis are common among adolescents, regular, heavy use is not. A systematic review of the literature on adolescent substance use and mental health symptomatology revealed a significant relationship between symptoms of depression and problematic substance use (Hussong et al., 2017). And a study of psychiatric symptoms among adolescents with a clinical diagnosis of substance use disorder (SUD) found that those with SUD were more likely to experience a higher intensity and variety of psychiatric symptoms than other adolescents. The authors suggest that adolescents identified as having problematic substance use should be referred to mental health treatment (Shrier et al., 2003). Additional research by Tapert et al.

(2001) showed that teens who meet the DSM criteria for alcohol or drug dependence are more likely to engage in risky sexual behavior.

Physical risks of substance use in adolescence

The most commonly used substances among adolescents are alcohol, tobacco, and cannabis (SAMHSA, 2021). And while overall, substance use is not common among young adolescents, the substances they choose have varying physical risks. Tobacco, for example, has a high rate of dependence and long-term physical consequences such as increased risk of lung cancer, chronic obstructive pulmonary disease (COPD), and emphysema. However, there is no risk of fatal overdose from tobacco use, therefore, harm reduction strategies can focus more on preventing regular adoption of tobacco and educating youth about the physical risks that can come on with longer term, frequent use. Because tobacco use can be hard to stop once started, special attention can be given to prevention.

Alcohol is another common substance used by adolescents. Like tobacco, alcohol use can be habit forming both physically and psychologically. Unlike tobacco, alcohol does present the risk of a fatal overdose. Harm reduction around alcohol includes not only information about the alcohol content in beer, wine, and liquor, but also how to recognize an alcohol overdose and what to do in that situation. Teens should be taught the symptoms of an alcohol overdose, how to prevent harms such as choking on vomit, or engaging in risky behavior, and should be encouraged to seek help for anyone exhibiting symptoms, even if the people in question are not of age to be drinking. Using punishment as a driver for prevention can backfire when it scares teens away from seeking help for fear of getting in trouble. Teens should always be encouraged to go to the hospital or medical facility when there is concern about a serious drug overdose. Many states have Good Samaritan Laws which exclude prosecution for illegal drug use for people seeking help for friends who are overdosing. However, not all state laws also include minors.

The rise in non-prescribed opiate use has raised concern for adolescents because it also poses the risk of fatal overdose. In 2022, an average of 22 high school students died of a drug overdose, and drug overdoses and poisonings are the third leading cause of preventable pediatric deaths in the United States (Friedman & Hadland, 2024). Beyond overdosing on opiates, this risk includes the ingestion of other substances like Fentanyl, which the teen may not be aware is in the product they are taking. A harm reduction strategy deployed to address tainted drugs is drug checking. Drug checking tests pills and powders for purity and tells the user if there are chemicals besides the ones they expect. Drug checking is important because it can prevent someone from taking a potentially dangerous substance or one that they do not intend on ingesting. Unfortunately, as we previously mentioned, drug checking stations have been outlawed from many festivals and other public events because of the RAVE Act (https://www.congress.gov/bill/108th-congress/senate-bill/226). Passed in 2003, the RAVE Act allowed concert promoters and party sponsors to be held criminally liable for drugs sold or consumed at their events. The presence of drug checking stations and other harm reduction services implies that promoters are aware of drug use at their events, so many promoters banned these services to prevent any implications that they have knowledge of drug use or drug selling.

When discussing the risk of fatal overdose from alcohol and opiates, it is important to bring up cannabis. There will be an entire section on cannabis later in this book. However, while cannabis does have some of the same habit forming qualities as tobacco, like tobacco, it also has no fatal overdose. THC, the psychoactive ingredient in cannabis, can be ingested at levels high enough to cause anxiety, overwhelming feelings, and sometimes panic. However, there is no level of THC that will cause death. During the years of cannabis prohibition, the nuances of safer cannabis use were not taught to teens. Rather, cannabis was lumped together with other illicit substances under the rhetoric of Just Say No. As a result, the true potential of cannabis and harm reduction was not explored. Because cannabis use cannot result in fatal overdose, some may argue that it is a better choice than alcohol or opiates for teens who are experimenting with intoxicating substances. While it is not harmless, death is a very serious and very permanent outcome. And while the overall message to teens is to delay all substance use as long as possible, part of a harm reduction approach is providing safety-based, nuanced information about the relative harms of different substances so that teens can make safer choices.

Adolescence is a time when the brain is continuing to mature. This impacts rational decision making and impulsive thinking. Not only can these impacts be related to the decisions to try substances and use them in risky situations, but the use of substances in a chronic and habitual way can impede brain development (Bava & Tapert, 2010). In recognition of the impact of early substance use on developing neuro-cognitive processes, programs like The Illicit Project aim to reduce use during this time period by using a neuro-science, harm reduction-based approach to reduce hazardous substance use and risky drug-related behaviors while increasing participant knowledge about how to reduce harm and increase safety. Based in Australia, The Illicit Project consists of three days of web-based programming and has an underlying strengths-based approach to instill in adolescents a desire to protect their brains during this time of vulnerability and developmental growth. The program uses a variety of interactive content to address peer resistance training, normative education, alcohol related harm reduction, the use of substances such as MDMA and cannabis, how to seek help when needed, and the impact that using substances has on them neurologically. A 2022 randomized controlled trial of The Illicit Project found that, compared to the control group, teens experiencing the program reported less binge drinking, monthly alcohol consumption, early onset cannabis use, risky cannabis or MDMA use, and nicotine use. The experimental group also reported experiencing fewer alcohol related harms and demonstrated a greater knowledge of drug use concepts in general (Debenham et al., 2022).

Psychological risks of substance use in adolescence

In addition to the physical risks of dependence and overdose, psychological risks exist as well. However this is a more complicated scenario because of the role of early childhood adverse events on both an increased likelihood of substance use and mental health issues. These are always related, but not necessarily interdependent. While there are teens who experience problematic substance use who have had no adverse experiences, and those who have mental health issues but do not use substances, the two are often intertwined. Making things even more complicated, there is a "chicken or egg" scenario where it can be tough to know which comes first.

Because of the panic felt by many parents at the thought of their teen engaging in substance use, focus is often on the substance itself, whether that be alcohol, tobacco, or cannabis. However, research suggests that, for early adolescent substance use, it is less about the substance and more about the establishment of a pattern of behavior that can escalate if not addressed. It is also suggested that the issue of poly substance use is important to address when noting this pattern of behavior. While substance use is rare in early adolescence, it often involves more than one substance and is predictive of issues later on (Moss, Chen, & Yi, 2014).

This is complicated by the role that early traumatic experiences have in both increasing the likelihood of hazardous substance use, but also the experience of mental health issues (Kirsch & Lippard, 2022).

The need to address psychological distress can occur before substances are an option. Part of harm reduction is identifying factors that may result in harm, and addressing them early, in a non-judgmental and supportive way. Because of the stigma that exists for kids who need counseling or additional support, parents may avoid these types of interventions with the hope that the issues will resolve themselves. Sometimes they do. But sometimes, kids with psychological disturbances become teens looking for ways to self-medicate and for peer groups that reflect their own struggles. We will discuss the impact of those peer groups more in the next section. While heavy, frequent use of intoxicating substances can lead to psychological distress, occasional substance use is unlikely to. This is why it is important, from a harm reduction perspective, to remove the judgment and fear, and look at behavior pragmatically. Is substance use occurring in the context of long exhibited symptoms of depression? A sudden upheaval like a divorce or death in the family? In conjunction with declining school performance or entry into a new peer group? In other words, beyond the substance use, what ELSE is happening and how are they related? Sometimes, addressing depression, divorce, school performance, and other personal and environmental factors will end up addressing the substance use as well. For young people, substance use is often more a symptom than a problem. Making it the focus can result in overlooking other psychological functioning issues that need attention. Hazardous or compulsive substance use can be indicative of a deeper mental health issue. Certain mental health conditions like depression, bipolar disorder, and ADHD, combined with substance use, can increase compulsivity and risk related behaviors (Welsh et al., 2020).

It should be noted, however, that regular, heavy use of psychoactive substances in adolescence can have a negative impact on psychosocial development independent of other life circumstances. During adolescence the brain is still developing, and centers that control rational thought and decision making are still being formed. Consistent and heavy use of substances during this time period can negatively impact this development. Going back to harm reduction, this is why use reduction is viewed as a positive step. If heavy use is a big risk factor for developmental interruption, succeeding in reducing the level of substance ingestion will reduce the chance for this potential harm. Thinking about it from the view of nutrition, a person who reduces their intake of fast food from seven times per week to two times per week will lessen the chance of harms related to ingesting fast food, even if they have not abstained completely. Reduction versus abstinence is tough for parents because of the "all use is abuse" trope. But, it is very much in line with starting where the client is, which is a key component of harm reduction.

Role of environmental and social factors in predicting, preventing, and addressing problematic substance use

As discussed in the research on the Gateway Theory, one risk factor for problematic substance use is the age of onset. The earlier a person tries an intoxicating substance, the greater their risk for not only substance progression, but hazardous use. But is this a case of nature or nurture? It is both. The early onset of substance use is related to both the genetic and psychological makeup of the individual, but also their environmental and social situation. As we like to say in social work, genetics loads the gun, but the environment pulls the trigger.

Scholars such as Harith Swadi (1999) have identified both internal and external factors for early initiation into substance use. In addition to risk factors, there exist protective factors that may stave off initiation until the teen is older and better able to handle the potential risks and impacts of substance use. From a genetic perspective, early initiation into substance use has been associated with personality attributes such as risk taking and a low level of harm avoidance. Environmental risk factors include the impact of peer groups and norms, and the presence or absence of traumatic life events and a chaotic home life. Teens who possess multiple risk factors including certain personality traits, peer influence and traumatic experiences are the most likely to not only engage in early substance use, but to participate in hazardous use. Beyond experimentation, it is this type of use that is more likely to result in dependence or other issues later on. The need to differentiate between experimentation and hazardous use as well as note the internal and external risk factors present is an important part of applying the techniques of harm reduction. Changing social roles also influence substance using behavior, especially changes in family roles such as those impacted by marriage, divorce, and economic instability (Staff et al., 2010).

Harm reduction is not only about substance use, but also improving the quality of peer and family relationships to reduce risk factors that influence behavior related to substances. The belief is that, by improving relationships, teens can make better decisions about their own health and well-being, including whether or not to use substances. Research supports that, while parental influence impacts substance using behavior throughout adolescence and into young adulthood, the nature of the influence changes. Parental monitoring is a protective factor in early adolescence. However, as teens mature, the impact of monitoring is superseded by an overall healthy parental relationship. One aspect of family therapy in the context of harm reduction, is to help the family members not only communicate, but set and respect boundaries. Healthy parental boundaries can establish parents as protective factors as teens age. One environmental component that remains a factor from adolescence into early adulthood is peer influence. The norms, values, and activities adopted by a peer group can influence the decision to use substances and to develop a lifestyle that includes them. Again, as we have mentioned, problematic substance use is usually a symptom of other issues in a teen's life, and the peers that they choose to hang around can be indicative of social, psychological, or physical manifestations of trauma or other risk factors (Van Ryzin, Fosco, & Dishion, 2012). Furthermore, many issues that might exacerbate adolescent substance use begin long before substances are an option, and, if left unattended can cause a cascade effect that results in the hazardous use of substances once they become available. This emphasizes the importance of engaging in family therapy as part of not only a treatment for adolescent substance use, but as a preventative measure (Otten et al., 2019). Rigter et al. (2013) conducted a randomized controlled trial of Multi-Dimensional Family Therapy (MDFT) to address heavy cannabis use by adolescents. The MDFT intervention was compared to individual psychotherapy. Although both interventions showed positive results, the MDFT outperformed the psychotherapy in the areas of treatment retention, cannabis dependence measures, and number of consumption days reported. MDFT incorporates the impact of influences from multiple areas of the adolescent's life as possibly contributing to harmful substance use.

Hazardous substance use among adolescents is complex because it is occurring during a time of rapid physical, psychological and developmental change. Thus, treatments that contain multiple components, including family therapy, as well as culturally relevant approaches have been the most successful (Fadus et al., 2019). One of the reasons it is important to differentiate between experimentation and problematic substance use is the ability to tailor appropriate treatment approaches. Interventions may not even need to address substance use if that use is not a contributing factor to the issue at hand. And, if substance use is problematic, other personal and family issues should be addressed as well. The ways in which we treat problematic adolescent substance use will not be the same as adults. And, moving past the "all use is abuse" assumption, allows for the discovery of the actual role that substance use is playing and the ways in which harm reduction and safety education can be implemented. In 2024, Welsh and colleagues conducted a literature review of interventions for adolescent substance use and made recommendations including the following principles: 1) the integration of care between substance use and mental health conditions with more emphasis on accessibility through schools, 2) the inclusion of Screening, Brief Intervention and Referral to Treatment (SBIRT) in treatment practices, 3) greater investment in social programs and family involvement in treatment, and 4) increased funding for harm reduction-based treatments.

Especially important in the discussion about the prevention of hazardous substance use among adolescents is the relationship between harm reduction and resilience. While harm reduction seeks to identify and control for environments and behaviors that might cause harm, a component of that is helping teens learn and use skills that assist them in navigating high-risk situations in a safer manner. These skills can be rooted in biological, psychological, or social behaviors, but all have an emphasis on equipping teens with the ability to make better and more informed decisions in the moment. Resiliency combined with harm reduction is a sound strategy when it comes to teens and substance use (Olsoon et al., 2003).

One of the places that most impacts a teen's sense of resiliency is school. Developing the skills necessary to navigate not only high-risk environments, but their own mental health and wellness has been linked to school engagement and social connectedness. Protective factors have been found to increase and decrease at different times throughout the school experience, declining through middle school and then increasing during high school (Kim et al., 2015). Research by Bond et al. (2007) explored this relationship and found that greater levels of social connectedness in secondary school was associated with lower levels of mental health symptoms and substance use post-secondary school. Furthermore, the social development model, which examines anti-social and pro-social outcomes has been shown to be a predictor of adolescent substance use (Catalano et al., 1996). One of the common outcomes for discovering that a teen is using substances is to remove them from school activities as punishment. As research suggests, this may exacerbate the problem by endangering their connectivity to school and pro-social activities. A 2003 longitudinal study by Bryant et al. analyzed data on 1897 adolescents from the Monitoring the Future Study. While school misbehavior and associating with peers who encourage misbehavior was connected to adolescent substance use, school bonding, effort, and achievement as well as parental support were negatively associated with teen substance use. This speaks to the need to address problematic teen substance use as part of a spectrum of positive and negative influences. As well as understanding potential underlying biological, psychological, and social influences on behavior. A harm reduction approach would suggest addressing the potential risks of the behavior and meeting the physical, mental, and social needs of the adolescent, but not necessarily using an approach that separates them from peers and school activities.

The school-family partnership is another potential focus for resiliency-based interventions focused on risk reduction and strengthening prevention. A randomized trial of the Resilient Families initiative in Melbourne, Australia, found that teens who participated in the initiative experienced a significant reduction in alcohol use compared to controls. The Resilient Families Initiative seeks to impact teen substance using behavior by strengthening the family relationship, educating teens on problem solving, conflict resolution and emotional awareness, and parents on youth culture, listening, communication, and drug and alcohol use. This model goes beyond the focus of substance use as the primary problem, and instead views hazardous substance use as a reaction to mental or emotional struggles. By teaching teens and their families tools for dealing with these struggles, they are reducing the likelihood of the teen using drugs or alcohol in a risky way in order to cope (Toumbourou et al., 2013).

The current barriers to implementing evidence informed prevention programs for teens include a lack of coordination and dissemination of research on evidence informed prevention strategies and program funding coming in small bursts rather than sustained, stable program specific support. A systematic review of the effectiveness of various interventions for adolescent substance use found that there is minimal research on programs aimed specifically at adolescents, and the researchers suggest that interventions designed for adults should be adapted and tested on the adolescent population. While there is evidence for the effectiveness of policies like taxation and age/advertising restrictions on reducing alcohol and tobacco use among teens, these interventions are not available for prohibited substances. And while harm reduction interventions like needle access and drug checking have shown a moderate to large effect for reducing risk in adults, these interventions have not been made available or tested in adolescent populations (Stockings et al., 2016). A 2007 systematic review by Toumbourou et al. of interventions for youth substance use found that prevention strategies aimed at school, family, and social-based vulnerabilities were successful, as well as harm reduction-based strategies for addressing teens engaging in risky substance use. But these findings need to result in a wider implementation of community-based prevention and harm reduction services. Additionally, there needs to be an increase in health professionals trained in prevention science who have accessed and learned from the evidence-based programs that exist. Programs should be community-specific and based on the needs of community members, which requires a robust method of assessing priority problems (Catalano et al., 2012; Steiker, 2008). A 2017 ethnographic study by Jenkins et al. analyzed interviews with 86 adolescents aged 13–18 as part of the Researching Adolescent Distress and Resilience study (RADAR). The participants were asked to describe their experiences with substances. Results supported the notion that adolescent substance use is deeply related to community context and greatly influenced by lived experiences. Harm reduction takes into account the influences of community on substance use related decision making, and also values the unique lived experiences of the adolescents involved, inviting them to be active participants in determining treatment plans and measures of success.

Even in light of the evidence supporting harm reduction-based programs, the United States has been slower to adopt such programs than other countries due to the moralistic views of substance use and the inability to see adolescent use as a spectrum that includes non-problematic use. A study of harm reduction stakeholders in Texas including PWUD, harm reductionists, and first responders found that PWUD are fearful of interacting with 911 and healthcare systems (Claborn et al., 2023). Teens who use substances may feel anxious about reaching out to adults for even basic safety information regarding substance use due to assumptions made about addiction and dependence, not to mention breaking the law.

Harm reduction programs focused on alcohol have had a greater level of acceptance in the United States given that alcohol use is legal and accepted for adults. Even so, although there is research to support moderate drinking goals versus abstinence for at-risk adolescents, adoption on a broad scale is difficult. Much of the research on harm reduction interventions for teens has been conducted outside of the U.S. Toumbourou et al. (2003) conducted a study on 3,300 Australian teens and found that, while alcohol use remains fairly stable throughout high school, increased drinking during senior year was associated with more harmful patterns after high school. The authors recommend a harm reduction-based strategy of reducing alcohol use from weekly to less than weekly to prevent this escalation.

There have been some harm reduction-based alcohol programs implemented in the U.S., but they are in need of long-term outcome studies. High school-based, alcohol focused harm reduction programs such as the Alcohol Misuse Prevention Study (AMPS), Risk Skills Training Programme (RSTP), and Life Skills Training Program have shown reductions in risky alcohol use and related behaviors for participants. However, more research is needed to determine how to maintain these gains in the long term (Neighbors et al., 2006; Marlatt & Witkiewitz, 2002). Another harm reduction focused alcohol intervention showing promising outcomes for young people is the Brief Alcohol Screening and Intervention for College Students (BASICS). This is a two-session program (assessment and feedback), with each session lasting 50 minutes. Rooted in motivational interviewing, the first BASICS session focuses on building rapport, assessment of current drinking behavior, and educating the participant on what constitutes a standard drink. The participant is then presented with a feedback report based on this information. The second session focuses on reviewing relevant alcohol information and the participant's feedback report. The goals of the program include the reduction of heavy drinking, hazardous drinking and related behaviors, and the increase in a realistic idea of how much the participant is drinking, how this level matches with average drinking behaviors of peers, and other physical, mental, and social determinants of the potential for alcohol related harms (e.g., a family history of alcohol abuse, gender differences) (Whiteside et al., 2010). Another study, a randomized clinical trial, mailed personal feedback to participants in response to reported drinking behaviors and assessments and also showed positive results in reducing harmful drinking behaviors (Larimer et al., 2007; Logan & Marlatt, 2010; Marlatt & Witkiewitz, 2010). Rather than focusing solely on abstinence, BASICS seeks to educate students about alcohol use, assess their current drinking patterns, and help them develop strategies for alcohol reduction and safety.

Legality, impacts on vulnerable communities, and collateral sanctions

Of course, there are more potential harms related to substance use than just the impacts of the drug itself. The prohibition of drugs and criminal penalties associated with their use can also be a cause of harm and enduring collateral sanctions in the life of an adolescent. As we discuss later, the rhetoric of the drug war has been infused into the policies and programs that shape healthcare and family services. Rather than support people looking to reduce the harm in their lives related to substance use, these systems more often take a paternalistic and punitive approach through mandatory drug testing as a requirement for services, mandated reporting, zero tolerance policies, and coerced treatment (Cohen et al., 2022). These system-based sanctions can be carried over into how parents address substance use with their teen. Parents often mimic the punitive-based approaches being taken by the larger healthcare and social service system. In many cases, school and home-based punishments for substance use include being dismissed from a team or group activity or isolated from peers. Unfortunately, while these approaches theorize that the experience of being kicked off a team will make a teen think twice about using drugs again, the effect is often the opposite. Peer connections and group activities are actually protective against problematic substance use. And while it is understandable to want a teen to stop hanging around with a peer group that normalizes substance use, great thought should be given to the impact of removing positive support systems from the teen's life in the name of punishment.

Beyond the school- and home-based punishments, the punitive treatment of substance use at all ages creates an opportunity for criminal justice involvement. We know that not all groups are treated equally when it comes to the War on Drugs. In 1986, the Anti-Drug Abuse Act created the 100-1 sentencing disparity between crack and powder cocaine. Then, in 1988, crack became the only drug where possession was deemed a federal crime. Additionally, discretionary sentencing by judges led to Black people being sentenced for twice as long for crack offenses than White people (National Association of Criminal Defense Lawyer, 2022). A 2020 report from the ACLU states that Black people are 3.6 times more likely to be arrested for marijuana than White people. And although, overall, penalties for marijuana are decreasing, since 2010, 31 states have seen increases in their racial disparities in marijuana arrests (ACLU, 2020). Human Rights Watch has compiled data around the racial disparities in drug policing. They have found that Black people comprise 62% of drug offenders admitted to state prison. And, in seven states, they make up between 80 and 90% of those sent to prison on drug charges. Nationwide, Black men are sent to state prison on drug charges at 13 times the rate of White men (Human Rights Watch, 2025). Of course, that was the goal of the War on Drugs in the first place. In 1994, Nixon's Domestic Policy Adviser, John Erlichman, said in an interview, "We knew we couldn't make it illegal to be either against the war or black, but by getting the public to associate the hippies with marijuana and blacks with heroin and then criminalizing them both heavily, we could disrupt those communities. We could arrest their leaders, raid their homes, break up their meetings, and vilify them night after night in the evening news. Did we know we were lying about the drugs? Of course we did" (Taifa, N., 2021).

The increased likelihood of arrest and lengthy sentencing for groups who already face educational and employment disparities creates a self-fulfilling prophecy around aspiration and success. Harm reduction is not just about methods for reducing personal harm, it encompasses the recognition of societal harm from the criminalization of drugs. Furthermore, the criminalization of drugs prevents harm reduction programs like syringe access and drug checking from being implemented, increasing the chance for personal harm and unsafe use. Considering harm reduction for adolescent substance use is both how we treat the use of drugs by adolescents and the policies we support that frame how drug use is treated by society.

The impacts of drug prohibition and the increased chance for criminal justice involvement has had far reaching and multi-generational impacts on some vulnerable communities. Research on the effects of parental incarceration show impact on attachment, stigma, physical and mental health, and the perpetuation of intergenerational trauma (Skinner-Osei, & Levenson, 2018). Additionally, the collateral sanctions associated with a drug arrest, including exclusion from federal college funding, encourages the further problematic use of substances tied to the experiences of depression and anxiety. Community trauma and its impact on individuals may also encourage substance use. Research by King et al. (2022) found depression, PTSD, and other traumas to be positive motivators for adolescent cannabis use, and that this was especially prevalent in the African American community, which has experienced a greater impact from drug prohibition than other communities.

Cannabis and psychedelics spotlight

While any substance use outside of a prescription medication is prohibited for adolescents, changes in cannabis policies and therapeutic use of both cannabis and psychedelics has resulted in a shift in how these substances are viewed and treated. During the Just Say No era of the 1980s and 1990s, teens were taught about alcohol in a way that gave them valuable information about how to use it safely. One ounce of liquor equals 4 ounces of wine equals 12 ounces of beer. The only thing that sobers you up is time. Don't drink and drive. What are the symptoms of alcohol poisoning? However, when it came to all other drugs, including cannabis and psychedelics, the message was only "Don't do it". So, how has the legalization of cannabis and the emergence of cannabis and psychedelics as therapeutic tools changed the conversation and the need for education, especially around harm reduction?

De-stigmatization

With legalization comes inevitable de-stigmatization. Part of the stigma against using cannabis and psychedelics came from the act of breaking the law. The other source of stigma came from stereotypes about who used these substances. Losers, burn outs, those with no ambition or respect for their parents. These were all images tied to the use of cannabis and psychedelics through programs like D.A.R.E., but also mainstream media, movies, and music. In the 1980s there was a PSA widely shown proclaiming "users are losers, and losers are users". And almost every sitcom from the era had a "very special episode" where something terrible befell a character who used drugs, with the main character barely escaping that fate by finally coming to their senses. This propaganda campaign against people who use drugs resulted in the notion that MOST people who use illegal drugs become addicted to them, when scientists like Carl Hart have shown that this just isn't true (Hart, 2013). So, what happens when a drug that we have invested so much time stigmatizing is not only legal, but being used by your grandma? This is the situation we find ourselves in when it comes to cannabis. The answer is actually taking a play from the alcohol playbook of the D.A.R.E. era: provide scientifically based, safety focused information for teens about these substances and how to reduce potential harm should they choose to use them.

Two programs that have emerged as harm reduction-based education on drugs are Know Drugs and Safety First. Know Drugs (https://knowdrugs.com/) works to not only educate teens about drug use, but in a way that provides actionable information on safety and risk reduction. Presenting drug use as a spectrum of behavior, the program also employs strategies drawn from real life scenarios that teens find themselves in, rather than the sitcom-ified stories we grew up with where the "bad" kid is the one who brings the drugs to the party and cajoles the "good" kids into going along. Safety First (https://drugpolicy.org/resource/safety-first/) is another drug education program rooted in science and harm reduction. First created by the Drug Policy Alliance, and now run by the Stanford REACH lab (https://med.stanford.edu/halpern-felsher-reach-lab/preventions-interventions/Safety-First.html), Safety First is focused on the principles of harm reduction and how they can be applied in a high school setting. The Stanford REACH lab has also developed a cannabis specific education curriculum also using harm reduction as a framework for educating teens about cannabis specifically. All of these programs seek to undo the harms of a Just Say No approach to substance use and instead introduce scientifically based information, safety techniques, and real life scenarios. As a direct response to the impacts that de-stigmatization may have on the appeal of cannabis and psychedelics, these programs also acknowledge that not all substance use is the same, even among adolescents. However even though cannabis is framed with less stigma, we are seeing cannabis use rates among adolescents decline, even post legalization. The reasoning for this may be related to who is using cannabis more often…their parents.

Observation of parental use

When we look back at the drug propaganda golden age of the 1980s and 1990s, another PSA that was commonly referenced involved a dad finding cannabis in his son's room. Upon asking him where he learned about smoking pot, the son hotly replied, "You! I learned it by watching you!" Thus was ingrained the idea that "parents who use drugs, have kids who use drugs". But is this assertion accurate? A 2018 study by Hill et al. looked at the relationship between parent and adolescent cannabis use with and without parental Cannabis Use Disorder. The results showed that the presence of CUD was predictive of adolescent cannabis use, but parental cannabis use without CUD was not. The study also showed that low positive parenting was a mediating factor between the presence of parental CUD and adolescent cannabis use, suggesting that it was not the cannabis use alone that was responsible for the adolescent use, but rather the resulting low positive parenting stemming from a parent's CUD. Seeing a parent use cannabis occasionally and non-problematically may not increase the chance of adolescent use, but the outcomes associated with problematic use might. To encourage a harm reduction approach to use, parents should not unnecessarily hide occasional cannabis use, but the preferred messaging supported by programs like Safety First is "delay". Explaining to teens that cannabis use is an adult activity and that it is something they should delay trying until they are older is a more realistic message than "Just Say No"…forever. Parents should, at the same time, educate teens on the safer use of cannabis and the impact that certain products, like those high in THC, can have on development. The point is not to scare them into abstinence, rather it is to present the ideal decision of "delay" but also arm their teen with information that will make their experience safer, should they choose to use cannabis. This approach also opens up a line of communication where teens feel comfortable coming to their parents with any concerns or questions they may have about cannabis.

Detangling medical versus recreational consumption

While much of cannabis and psychedelics use is for recreational purposes, these substances also have proven therapeutic value and are being used more and more commonly to treat pain, depression, anxiety, and insomnia as well as medical conditions like PTSD, multiple sclerosis, and Parkinson's disease. For people who use cannabis and psychedelics as medicine, use may be more frequent and intense than a joint on the weekends while watching a movie. In these cases, teens should be educated the way they would around any other medication being used by their parents. This fits into a broader harm reduction conversation about not using medications that are prescribed for other people, including cannabis and psychedelics. Medications are meant specifically for those they are prescribed and using other people's medications whether it be cannabis, Oxy, or Adderall can result in harm. This does not mean that the conversation around medical use of cannabis and psychedelics should not include safety information about use and risk, just that the message concerning the use of other people's medications should be included. Teens are old enough to understand this message, while younger children may simply be looking to mimic the actions of their parents, which is why all medications, including cannabis and psychedelics, should be kept locked up and out of reach.

Occasionally the teen themselves may be the one using cannabis or psychedelics for therapeutic purposes. Childhood conditions like cancer, autism, and other behavioral issues may benefit from the use of these substances. Teens who are using them medicinally should be educated about the importance of not sharing them with friends and that their use of them is the same as the use of any other medications. They should take them only as directed and let their parents know of any unwanted side effects.

Parents may feel uneasy talking to their teens about cannabis and psychedelics. Their own use and the continued stereotyping of users as "losers" may make harm reduction focused conversations seem phony and inauthentic. If a parent discovers that their teen has used cannabis, even if it is legal for adults and they themselves use it, their first instinct may be punitive and to support the "all use is abuse" narrative. They may bring their teen to a professional with fears that use is indicative of something more serious. In these scenarios, a professional can support these conversations by keeping them factually accurate and safety focused. See Exercise 2: Cannabis and harm reduction in an age of legalization, for more on working with young people around cannabis in an era of policy change.

Chapter 5

Drug Policy's Impact on Addiction Treatment and Drug Education

Drug policies are public health measures that include a set of laws and regulations that direct the control, distribution, use, and treatment of drugs within a culture. They are supposed to balance public safety, health, social justice, and individual freedoms, and reflect the values and priorities of a society. Drugs can be divided into *licit* – those legally permitted and regulated (e.g., alcohol and prescription drugs) – or *illicit* (e.g., heroin and cocaine), which are illegal and usually prohibited. Both types can carry risks of misuse and health consequences, but only illicit drugs are usually criminalized.

As we reviewed in Chapter 1, the War on Drugs and its attendant policies have played, and continue to play, a predominant role in shaping both the development of and access to addiction treatment in the United States. We begin this section by examining how drug policy has directly contributed to adolescent overdose risk, particularly by limiting access to accurate drug education, harm reduction resources, and evidence-based care. The sections that follow build on this discussion by exploring how these policies have trickled down into the treatment landscape, shaping clinical practices, institutional norms, and public perceptions, and how harm reduction-informed approaches have emerged in response, offering more adaptive and compassionate options for adolescents and their families.

Drug Policy and Adolescent Overdose Risk

In their 2024 *New England Journal of Medicine* article, Friedman and Hadland present a compelling analysis of the urgent and ongoing public health challenge of adolescent overdose in the United States. They note that while adolescent drug use has declined, overdose deaths have more than doubled since 2019, largely due to the proliferation of counterfeit pills containing illicit fentanyl, often resembling prescription medications and appealing to adolescents who may be experimenting, self-medicating trauma, or unsuspecting of the risk.

Importantly, Friedman and Hadland challenge traditional narratives rooted in drug war ideology – particularly those that frame substance use as a moral failing or individual weakness – by emphasizing that most adolescent overdose deaths are unintentional and involve youth without a diagnosed opioid use disorder (OUD). This reframing highlights how many young people who die from overdose are not chronic or dependent users, but rather teens who may be experimenting, self-medicating, or unaware of the risks – especially in the context of a drug supply contaminated by illicit fentanyl. This observation disrupts common assumptions that overdose only occurs among "addicts", and instead reveals the broader harms caused by a punitive framework that focuses on moral judgment and criminalization rather than prevention, education, and care.

DOI: 10.4324/9781003581857-6

The article underscores the urgent need for widespread harm reduction education, including accurate information about fentanyl, counterfeit pills, and overdose response training, and low-barrier access to evidence-based treatment options, such as medications for OUD. This includes strategies like naloxone access in schools, social media outreach tailored to youth, and replacing fear-based messaging with honest, developmentally appropriate communication. It also emphasizes the importance of equipping adolescents, their caregivers, and the adults who support them, such as parents, educators, and healthcare providers, with the tools, training, and resources necessary to recognize risk, respond effectively, and access appropriate care without fear of punishment or stigma. They emphasize that effective prevention must address mental health, social determinants, and racial and geographic disparities. Notably, they call attention to the fact that only 11% of adolescents who died of overdose had ever received substance use treatment, pointing to systemic barriers and the urgent need to expand access to evidence-based interventions, such as buprenorphine, in settings that work with and support youth.

Good Samaritan laws are state-level policies designed to reduce the legal barriers that prevent people from calling for help during an overdose. These laws typically offer some degree of legal protection from arrest or prosecution for certain low-level drug offenses (such as possession or paraphernalia) when someone seeks emergency assistance for themselves or another person experiencing an overdose. However, protections vary significantly across states. In some cases, Good Samaritan laws do not extend to minors, do not protect the person who overdosed, or are written in ways that make their scope unclear. This inconsistency can lead to confusion and hesitation among adolescents, who may fear getting in trouble or putting someone else at risk by calling for help. The Prescription Drug Abuse Policy System (PDAPS) provides a helpful interactive map and dataset detailing these laws state by state, making it easier to understand how protections differ across jurisdictions (Center for Public Health Law Research, 2023).

Naloxone access laws are designed to complement Good Samaritan protections by ensuring that community members – not just healthcare professionals – can legally obtain and administer naloxone, a medication that rapidly reverses opioid overdoses. These laws often allow pharmacists to dispense naloxone without a patient-specific prescription, permit statewide standing orders, and provide legal immunity for laypersons who administer the drug in good faith. As with Good Samaritan laws, naloxone access policies also differ widely between states. The Network for Public Health Law offers a comprehensive 50-state legal survey that tracks key features of naloxone access laws, such as third-party prescribing and standing orders (Network for Public Health Law, 2023).

Together, Good Samaritan and naloxone access laws reduce both the fear and the helplessness that often surround overdose events. One protects the act of calling for help; the other provides the tools to intervene effectively. But for these laws to be truly effective, adolescents, families, educators, and healthcare providers must be informed about their rights and responsibilities. Bystander training and overdose education – integrated into schools, youth programs, and clinical settings – can empower young people to act quickly and confidently, shifting the response to overdose from fear and avoidance to care and connection.

Drug Policy and Access to Evidence-Based Care

Despite decades of evidence supporting harm reduction approaches, most addiction treatment providers in the United States continue to prioritize abstinence-based models and fail to integrate harm reduction into their services (Abraham et al., 2020; White, 2014).

Many programs remain deeply influenced by 12-step philosophies, which often reject harm reduction as "enabling" rather than recognizing its effectiveness in engaging individuals across stages of change (Marlatt et al., 2012). As Vakharia (2024) argues in *The Harm Reduction Gap*, this exclusion is not accidental – it reflects the enduring influence of drug war ideologies that frame abstinence as morally superior and marginalize public health strategies that center autonomy and care. This disconnect between research and practice is particularly stark in adolescent residential treatment.

In a national study, King et al. (2023) identified a troubling gap between clinical best practices and the services actually provided: although buprenorphine is FDA-approved for adolescents aged 16 and up and widely regarded as a gold standard for OUD, only 24.4% of facilities offered it, and just 10.6% provided ongoing treatment. Some programs even required teens to taper off buprenorphine before admission. While most facilities employed psychiatric prescribers and stocked naloxone, fewer than half included families in care, and many relied on non-evidence-based interventions like equine therapy, which, revealingly, was more common than buprenorphine access.

This fragmented and inconsistent treatment landscape leaves families with the burden of navigating a system shaped more by ideology than by science. Based on King et al.'s study, the average parent may need to call nine different programs just to locate one that offers developmentally appropriate, evidence-based care – assuming they have the time, resources, and knowledge to do so. Despite decades of evidence supporting buprenorphine and other effective treatments, accessible, evidence-based options for youth remain limited, especially for those who are low-income, uninsured, or from marginalized communities. We frequently encounter situations in our work with teens where the right tools exist, but the system fails to provide them. This disconnect leaves us feeling disheartened because our clients and their families are left without meaningful options and underscores how treatment access is still shaped more by outdated policies and ideology than by science or public health priorities. These gaps reflect the lasting imprint of drug war ideologies that prioritize abstinence and punishment over public health and equity.

Drug Policy Narratives

A helpful way to understand drug policy's direct impact on families seeking addiction treatment is by reviewing the various public health *narratives* – the stories that shape how health issues are understood, communicated, and addressed in a society. These narratives provide a specific lens through which health concerns are viewed, and thereby can influence public perception, policy-making, and individual behavior. Drug policy narratives shape social attitudes which in turn affects how individuals seek and receive treatment for addiction.

The sidebar highlights key drug policy narratives that continue to shape how substance use is perceived and treated.

The War on Drugs narrative: The War on Drugs has functioned as a broader war on people, particularly those from marginalized communities, by framing substance use as a criminal issue rather than a public health concern. This punitive framework has deeply influenced addiction treatment, often diverting funding away from health-based services and into criminal justice interventions. As a result, many one-size-fits-all treatment programs became integrated into or mandated by the legal system (e.g., drug courts), prioritizing abstinence and compliance over individualized care. Crucially, the narrative ignores the reality that drugs themselves are inanimate objects – neutral substances whose impact depends on the context of use, the individual, and their environment. By treating the drug as the enemy, rather than addressing the complex social, psychological, and structural factors that shape substance use, the War on Drugs has pathologized and punished people instead of supporting them. The war's legacy includes the stigmatization of drug users and their families, contributing to widespread mistrust of treatment systems and deterring help-seeking behaviors. Today, this stigma remains a powerful barrier, especially for families who fear judgment, legal consequences, or child welfare involvement when trying to access support.

Prohibition and criminalization narrative: As a corollary to the War on Drugs narrative, this narrative demonizes drugs and drug users, and views use as a moral failing or criminal activity, advocating for legal penalties rather than treating it as a health issue. Policies rooted in criminalization are based on prohibiting the use of substances, often prioritize incarceration over treatment, exacerbate social stigma, marginalize substance users, and can create barriers to future well-being. Prohibition's extensive reach has infiltrated and become ingrained in predominant prevention education models – such as the "Just Say No" campaign (see Chapter 2) – 12-step mutual help groups (AA, NA), and the addiction treatment industry's one-size-fits-all, abstinence-only model. As a result of the prevailing treatment model embracing a prohibition narrative, the person-centric, compassionate, science- and health-based treatments used with every other mental health and medical condition are often ignored.

The All or Nothing Narrative: This prohibition mindset carries over into most traditional treatment models, where recovery is framed as an all-or-nothing pursuit, with total abstinence as the only acceptable outcome. Much like prohibitionist policies, like alcohol prohibition in the 1920s (Chapter 2), that have historically ignored harm reduction strategies in favor of punitive measures, abstinence-only treatment often prioritizes rigid ideology over practical, life-saving interventions. For teens, who are often exploring, experimenting, and navigating peer influences, this rigid model can feel particularly out of touch with their realities, pushing them away from support rather than toward it. Emphasizing abstinence as the primary measure of success often requires individuals to count their "recovery" time in days of sobriety. In spaces like AA and NA meetings, a single instance of drug use is labeled as a relapse, forcing individuals to reset their progress back to zero. This rigid perspective fosters a culture of secrecy, where individuals may hide their struggles due to the fear of judgment and consequences. Unfortunately, this secrecy can have dangerous consequences, particularly when people experience a setback after a period of abstinence. Reduced tolerance and exposure to potent substances like fentanyl can lead to fatal overdoses – situations that might have been prevented if individuals felt safe to seek help. The shame and failure associated with slips also discourage people from attempting treatment again, as they may feel disheartened by unrealistic standards of success.

Medicalization and Disease Model narrative: This narrative presents the perspective of addiction as a chronic progressive disease similar to diabetes or hypertension. An important benefit of medicalization of addiction has led to the development of medication-assisted treatment (e.g., buprenorphine, suboxone, and naltrexone) and evidence-based therapies to treat substance use disorders (SUDs). However, the negative consequences of this narrative have also led to a reliance on pharmaceutical interventions, ignoring crucial psychosocial supports that are part of a more comprehensive approach. An unintended consequence of medicalization is that it excessively relies on diagnoses which can reinforce stigma by "labeling" adolescents who use substances as "addicts". To explore this further, see Chapter 10, which examines how stigmatizing SUD diagnoses often overlook the mental health and psychosocial factors underlying a teen's struggles.

Courts as Gatekeepers narrative: Drug courts were originally introduced as a reform-minded alternative to incarceration, intended to address substance-related offenses through treatment rather than punishment. However, instead of shifting control to the healthcare system, they have reinforced the criminal justice system's authority over addiction by embedding medical decision-making within legal oversight. In this legal-medical hybrid system, judges – often without medical or psychiatric training – routinely impose treatment plans, approve or deny medication-assisted treatment (MAT), and define "successful" recovery based on legal compliance rather than clinical assessment (Sousa, 2021). Many courts continue to prohibit or limit access to evidence-based treatments like methadone and buprenorphine, favoring abstinence-only models despite medical consensus on the efficacy of MAT for opioid use disorder (Matusow et al., 2013). These practices reflect a persistent belief that coercion leads to recovery, and they compel individuals into rigid, one-size-fits-all programs that often disregard co-occurring mental health needs, trauma histories, and personal readiness for change. While drug courts are often framed as compassionate alternatives, they continue to criminalize substance use and punish relapse – a predictable part of recovery – with extended supervision or incarceration. The result is a system that prioritizes obedience over health, deepens involvement with the legal system, and raises serious ethical concerns about due process, medical autonomy, and the right to appropriate care.

In Chapter 4 we described the concerns with Just Say No educational programs which reinforce all of the above narratives. The Safety First alternatives mentioned acknowledge the harm reduction tenet that the drugs themselves aren't the problem, but a person's relationship with them and how they are used can be problematic.

Public Health-Oriented Drug Policies

Over time, in response to the shortcomings of prohibition and the War on Drugs, narratives have shifted somewhat, moving from punitive, prohibition-based frameworks to more health-centered, public health, social justice, and harm reduction-informed approaches. Recognizing that some individuals may not be able to abstain but can still reduce associated health risks, public health-related narratives shift the focus to health and social well-being, framing addiction as a public health and social justice issue. These narratives acknowledge that the impact of harmful drug policies and addiction are not distributed equally, often disproportionately affecting marginalized and minority communities. This framework opens the door to a wider array of treatment options, including methadone maintenance, needle exchange programs, and overdose prevention centers.

Some large urban areas, like New York City, Chicago, Los Angeles, Philadelphia, and Seattle have implemented public health-oriented drug policies that are harm reduction-based (National Harm Reduction Coalition, https://harmreduction.org/). They promote community engagement, culturally relevant interventions, counseling, supervised substance use interventions, and mental health services, and provide parents with supportive options. These policies reduce the risk of legal penalties and encourage parents to seek help without fearing punitive consequences for their adolescents. In some communities parents can also participate in harm-reduction training and community support groups, empowering them to approach their teen's behavior more constructively (Partnership to End Addiction, n.d.).

Community programs play a vital role in supporting families affected by substance use by creating safe, inclusive spaces for connection, guidance, and resilience-building. One example is HRH413 (Harm Reduction Hedgehogs 413), a peer-led harm reduction organization in Western Massachusetts founded by Jess Tilley and Albie Park. Through street outreach, HRH413 reaches individuals who may not access traditional syringe services, with a focus on serving marginalized populations such as people of color and transgender individuals. The organization also facilitates Harm Reduction Works (HRW), a mutual help group open to people who use drugs as well as family members, friends, and allies. HRW offers a flexible, nonjudgmental alternative to abstinence-only models, promoting education, safer strategies, and community support for all those impacted by substance use (Harm Reduction Hedgehogs, n.d.). Social justice-oriented drug policies focus on reducing disparities in access to treatment and support. For parents from marginalized communities, these policies can improve access to resources, offer culturally appropriate support, and reduce the potential for discriminatory treatment in schools and healthcare settings.

Prohibition-Based Drug Policy Impact on Families and Parenting

Policies that prioritize criminalization and punitive responses versus the rehabilitation and supportive services of harm reduction dramatically impact how parents navigate their adolescent's substance use. For example, the zero-tolerance for any drug use that these policies require often creates an environment of family fear and secrecy, with parents hesitant to seek help due to the risk of legal consequences for their teen. This can lead to increased stress and tension within families, where parents may feel isolated or stigmatized. Zero-tolerance approaches are reinforced via the parent education and messaging from 12-step mutual help groups (Al-Anon) and addiction rehabs.

Much of this messaging stems from the widespread "tough love" myth, which promotes the idea that parents should manage adolescent substance use through control and punishment rather than open communication. This approach stands in direct contrast to the research on authoritative parenting, which supports warmth, structure, and dialogue as protective factors (see Chapter 9). When parents are encouraged to take a punitive stance, trust and communication can erode, creating conditions that not only hinder adolescent development but also increase the risk of more problematic substance use and disengagement from support. These dynamics run counter to the goals of harm reduction, which emphasize connection, collaboration, and individualized care. When people are told they must not do something, they often experience psychological reactance – a psychological resistance to perceived threats against personal autonomy. Originally developed by Brehm (1966) and expanded by Wicklund (1974), reactance theory explains how restrictions on freedom evoke emotional arousal and efforts to regain control. Brehm and Brehm (1981) later integrated these ideas into a broader framework that continues to inform how we understand resistance, especially in mandated contexts.

Given that adolescent brain development is still ongoing, we recommend abstinence – or at the very least, delaying substance use – as the safest approach, since later initiation is associated with better outcomes (see Chapter 9). At the same time, the harm reduction principle of meeting teens where they are becomes essential. As discussed in Chapter 9, expecting strict abstinence or using coercive strategies often backfires, leading to increased resistance, secrecy, or higher-risk use. These approaches conflict with what we know about adolescent development and can ultimately result in more harm than good.

Prohibition-Based Drug Policy Impact on Schools and Communities

In school districts with strict zero-tolerance policies, adolescents caught using drugs may face expulsion or academic penalties. Even for students who struggle academically, attending school provides an important daily structure and routine as well as beneficial peer and interpersonal interactions. Participation in extracurricular activities like athletics, band, and after-school clubs, are important to developing a healthy purpose in life and bolstering self-esteem. Removal from school adds significant pressure on parents to manage both academic and behavioral support for their teens. Additionally, expulsion from school limits access to health services and programs, and can result in disrupted academic progress. It stigmatizes families and parents, making it difficult for them to access community resources and parents may feel blamed for their adolescent's behavior.

Many school districts implement Student Assistance Programs (SAPs) as an early intervention strategy for students perceived to be at risk for mental health challenges and substance use. These programs have the potential to provide valuable resources, counseling, and support to students struggling with emotional distress or experimenting with substances. However, SAPs often rely on Just Say No-style prevention efforts, which emphasize abstinence-based messaging rather than nuanced, safety and evidence-based approaches. These programs may frame all substance use as equally dangerous, failing to differentiate between casual experimentation and problematic use – a distinction that is crucial for effective intervention.

One significant concern with SAPs is the one-size-fits-all nature of some of their interventions. In many cases, students identified as "at-risk" may be required to attend mandatory addiction treatment programs, even when they have not developed a substance use disorder (SUD) or when their substance use is a symptom of underlying mental health issues that remain unrecognized and untreated. Worse, placing students with mild or experimental substance use into therapy groups alongside peers with severe addiction issues can exacerbate risks rather than mitigate them. Research suggests that grouping lower-risk youth with those who engage in more severe substance use can lead to peer reinforcement of problematic behaviors, increasing rather than reducing the likelihood of future substance misuse (Dishion et al., 1999).

A sometimes-devastating consequence of punitive, prohibition-based policies in education is the development of the *school-to-prison pipeline* – the process by which students, particularly those from marginalized communities, are pushed out of educational environments and into the criminal justice system. Central to this pipeline are zero-tolerance policies that rely on exclusionary discipline practices such as suspensions and expulsions, and the growing presence of law enforcement officers in schools (Wald & Losen, 2023). As the Center for Public Justice (n.d.) describes, this shift has led to a form of "mission creep" where schools increasingly adopt punitive measures that criminalize student behavior rather than support development. These environments disproportionately affect students who already face academic, behavioral, or social challenges, reinforcing existing cycles of inequality, poverty, and incarceration.

Removing students from their learning environments – whether through exclusionary discipline or through criminal justice involvement – can severely disrupt academic progress and increase the likelihood of dropping out. Students who are expelled, suspended, or referred to juvenile detention are often funneled into under-resourced alternative programs or removed from school entirely, making reintegration difficult. The Center for Public Justice also cites data showing that the presence of school resource officers correlates with higher suspension rates, particularly for drug-related infractions, which compounds these risks. These disciplinary disparities are especially pronounced for Black and Latine students, who are more likely to be targeted by harsh enforcement practices. Ultimately, the long-term consequences can include limited access to higher education, employment barriers, and an increased likelihood of future incarceration.

In response to concerns about exclusionary discipline, harm reduction-oriented strategies provide a thoughtful alternative to more punitive approaches in schools. To reduce the impact of the school-to-prison pipeline, the Education Law Center in Philadelphia (n.d.), advocates for restorative practices that emphasize conflict resolution, relationship-building, and accountability. These include using peer mediation circles in place of suspension, embedding school-based mental health professionals to address behavioral needs, and replacing school resource officers with trained behavioral support staff.

Community-led initiatives – such as those led by the Dignity in Schools Campaign (n.d.) – further illustrate the power of grassroots reform. These movements prioritize care, equity, and inclusion over surveillance and punishment, and emphasize the importance of student voice in shaping safer and more just school environments. Together, these efforts call for a systemic reevaluation of how we define school safety and success – moving away from control-based models toward approaches rooted in trust, support, and community accountability.

Prohibition-Based Myths about Addiction and Treatment

Within the traditional SUD provider community, however, science-based parenting approaches have often been subverted by parenting "advice" based on prohibition-based myths, such as "tough love", the need to "hit bottom", "enabling", and the cannabis "gateway" to more dangerous drugs. These are myths because they are based on prohibition narratives with little to no research to support them. When confronted with the reality that their teen is using drugs in an unsafe manner, it's natural for parents to be very frightened and confused about appropriate steps to take. They can often feel under siege and disempowered by the one-size-fits-all mutual-help groups' advice and providers' recommendations that can have deleterious outcomes if this advice is taken. Harm reduction parenting empowers parents by encouraging them not to ignore their instincts and knowledge about their unique family circumstances (Lessin, 2023a).

Taking a closer look at the myths will help understand the contrasts between the myths and science-based harm reduction approaches, and shed some light on strategies for parents and families to take in intervening with their child's substance use.

"Being ready" for treatment/hitting bottom

The concept of "being ready" to enter treatment for substance use is often framed as a necessary precondition for change, suggesting that people must reach a point of crisis or personal reckoning before they can successfully modify their substance use. This idea is closely tied to the "hitting bottom" narrative, which assumes that significant pain, loss, or consequences are required to motivate change. In many traditional treatment models, particularly those influenced by 12-step programs, readiness is seen as something that emerges only after a person has endured enough suffering to recognize the need for help. This perspective can lead to a wait-and-see approach in which interventions and support are withheld until someone is deemed "ready".

Rather than waiting for a crisis, harm reduction provides low-barrier, non-coercive options – such as safer use strategies, overdose prevention, or medication-assisted treatment – that allow people to make incremental changes on their own terms. This approach shifts the focus from forcing readiness through suffering to creating supportive conditions that empower people to make choices at their own pace, reducing harm and increasing the likelihood of sustainable change. While some may find motivation for change through hardship, others benefit from incremental steps and non-coercive support, highlighting the value of diverse approaches to substance use and behavior change.

The Stages of Change Model (SOC), also known as the Transtheoretical Model (Prochaska & DiClemente, 1983), outlines how individuals move through different phases of behavior change, particularly in addressing substance use. This model challenges the traditional notion that change only occurs after a person "hits bottom". Instead, it recognizes that change is a process, not a single event, and that individuals can engage in meaningful behavior shifts at any stage. SOC accounts for adolescents' unique developmental process by recognizing that their motivation, decision-making, and behavior shifts are often nonlinear, influenced by external pressures, social dynamics, and ongoing brain maturation, requiring flexible, engagement-focused interventions rather than rigid treatment expectations. Chapter 10 provides a fuller examination of the stages of change.

A growing body of research challenges the assumption that formal treatment or conscious readiness is always necessary for change. Longitudinal studies such as the National Epidemiologic Survey on Alcohol and Related Conditions (NESARC) have shown that a significant percentage of individuals with substance use disorders reduce or stop using substances without formal intervention. This phenomenon, sometimes referred to as "maturing out", suggests that for many, especially adolescents and young adults, behavior change often unfolds gradually as part of a broader developmental process.

Adolescents may reduce risky substance use as a result of neurodevelopmental maturation, evolving priorities, and life transitions, such as entering work, forming intimate relationships, or pursuing education. Improvements in impulse control, emotional regulation, and future-oriented thinking contribute to healthier decision-making over time. For many, this shift happens organically rather than through deliberate efforts to quit. While external pressures – such as family expectations, school mandates, or legal consequences – may push youth into treatment before they feel internally motivated, change can still emerge over time. Importantly, not all risky behaviors in adolescence reflect a chronic condition requiring intensive treatment; many are developmentally normative and tend to resolve without formal intervention. Recognizing this allows us to shift the clinical stance from one of forcing readiness to one of creating developmentally attuned support that honors the adolescent's evolving capacity for growth and change (Peele & Brodsky, 1991). At the same time, this perspective should not diminish the value of formal treatment, which remains vital for many adolescents, particularly those facing co-occurring mental health concerns, structural vulnerabilities, or chronic patterns of use.

Tough love

The tough love philosophy has played a significant role in shaping coercive treatment models, particularly within the adolescent residential treatment industry. Rooted in the belief that strict discipline, forced confrontation, and harsh consequences will "break" a young person's resistance to change, tough love has been used to justify coercive, punitive, and often abusive interventions. Programs influenced by this approach – including many "troubled teen" residential centers, boot camps, and behavior modification facilities – have been criticized for employing physical restraint, emotional degradation, and isolation, and forcing teens into treatment against their will, often through "secure transport" services that forcibly remove them from their homes (Szalavitz, 2006).

Using tough love can profoundly harm families by severing vital connections between parents and children at a time when support is most needed. When parents are encouraged to cut off contact, impose harsh ultimatums, or expel their child from the home, the intended lesson of accountability can backfire, leading to isolation, increased risk, and deeper entrenchment in harmful behaviors. Tough love operates on the belief that a child must face the full consequences of their actions alone, yet in reality, it can damage or even destroy a child's life-sustaining connection to the only people who truly care.

In cases where there is no violence or abuse in the home, removing a child from their family environment can be disastrous, leaving them vulnerable to homelessness, exploitation, and untreated mental health issues. Research shows that youth who experience family rejection or are forced out of their homes face significantly higher rates of substance-related harm, depression, and suicide risk (Ryan et al., 2009). Rather than promoting positive change, tough love often reinforces shame and alienation, making it harder for young people to seek support or envision a path forward. In contrast, harm reduction approaches emphasize maintaining connection, setting compassionate boundaries, and providing a stable foundation for growth, recognizing that lasting change is more likely when a person feels safe and supported.

Enabling

Traditional definitions of enabling, particularly within 12-step and tough love frameworks, suggest that any form of support that does not enforce abstinence encourages continued substance use. This perspective assumes that pain and consequences are the primary motivators for change, leading families to withhold resources, cut off contact, or impose strict ultimatums – even when doing so increases risk. In these frameworks, parents who continue to offer emotional or material support may be told they are preventing their child from "hitting bottom" and interfering with recovery.

Harm reduction challenges this narrative by rejecting the idea that support inherently causes harm. It distinguishes between harmful enabling and compassionate support, recognizing that providing a loved one with food, housing, or emotional connection does not encourage substance use but helps prevent the life-threatening consequences of instability, trauma, and isolation. Rather than viewing care as a barrier to change, harm reduction sees maintaining relationships, reducing harm, and offering safer alternatives as essential. Instead of forcing individuals into crisis, harm reduction empowers families to set boundaries while still providing support, allowing for self-directed, sustainable change.

The stigma of enabling places parents in an impossible position: follow their instincts to nurture and protect, or risk being shamed as part of the problem. In 12-step communities, parents who do not embrace tough love may be judged as weak or failing to set firm enough boundaries, wearing the label of "enabler" as a badge of shame. Yet withholding support can increase harm, pushing young people toward homelessness, survival-based risk-taking, and deeper substance use. Harm reduction challenges this false dichotomy by arguing that love and support are not the problem – harm and risk are. Instead of forcing families into rigid, all-or-nothing choices, harm reduction encourages a balanced approach, allowing parents to offer compassionate, practical support while prioritizing their own well-being.

Gateway theory

Though previously discussed in Chapter 3, the gateway theory – the idea that cannabis use inevitably leads to the use of harder drugs–deserves a brief revisit here in light of its ongoing impact on parental beliefs and approaches to adolescent drug use. This theory is a legacy of prohibition-era drug policy rather than science, and its endurance reflects a widespread misunderstanding of adolescent substance use. Although early use can be one of many risk markers, research consistently shows that most teens who try cannabis do not progress to more dangerous substances. Still, this myth contributes to amplifying parental fear, often distracting from more relevant concerns such as patterns of use, co-occurring mental health issues, or harm-reduction strategies. The author spends a considerable amount of time in family therapy sessions helping parents unpack this misconception, offering evidence-based education so they can respond to their teen's behavior with more clarity and less fear.

Words Have Meaning: How the Drug War Shapes the Language We Use

Language plays a crucial role in shaping perceptions, influencing policy, and impacting the self-worth of individuals, particularly when discussing PWUD. The phrase "words have meaning" underscores how the language we use – whether intentionally or unknowingly – can either perpetuate stigma or foster understanding and support. Stigmatizing terms like "addict", "alcoholic", "junkie", or "substance abuser" reduce individuals to their drug use, reinforcing harmful stereotypes that suggest moral failure, criminality, or hopelessness. These labels contribute to discrimination, discourage people from seeking help, and reinforce punitive policies rather than compassionate, evidence-based approaches to substance use.

By shifting to person-first, non-stigmatizing language, such as "person who uses drugs" (PWUD), "people with an addiction", or "person experiencing substance use disorder", we acknowledge the individual beyond their drug use, reinforcing dignity and the possibility of change. Research shows that language shapes not only public attitudes but also the way healthcare professionals and policymakers respond to substance use. Using compassionate, accurate language can help break down barriers to care, reduce shame, and promote harm reduction approaches that prioritize health and well-being over punishment. Recognizing the power of words is an essential step in creating more effective, person-centered responses to substance use.

Saying "drug misuse" instead of "drug abuse" is important because it reduces stigma, acknowledges complexity, and aligns with a health-centered approach rather than a moralistic one. The word "abuse" carries negative connotations of wrongdoing, criminality, and moral failure. It suggests intentional harm and often leads to blame and punishment rather than support. In contrast, "misuse" recognizes that drug use exists on a spectrum and that people may use substances in ways that are harmful without meaning to cause harm (e.g., taking more than prescribed, using in unsafe situations). Shifting from "abuse" to "misuse" helps frame substance use as a public health issue rather than a moral failing, encouraging compassion, treatment, and evidence-based interventions rather than stigma and punishment. The words "clean" and "dirty" are problematic when referring to substance use because they reinforce stigma, moral judgment, and shame. Saying someone is "clean" after stopping drug use implies that when they were using, they were "dirty", which dehumanizes them and suggests that drug use makes a person morally impure or unworthy. This kind of language can create shame and guilt, discouraging people from seeking help or engaging with harm reduction services for fear of being judged.

Instead, neutral, non-stigmatizing language should be used, such as "substance-free" or "in recovery" instead of "clean", and "positive" or "negative" for drug tests instead of "dirty". These terms are factual and do not attach moral value to a person's substance use status. Language should reflect respect and dignity, reinforcing that a person's worth is not defined by their drug use. Using words like "recovery" and "relapse" can be problematic because they are often tied to abstinence-based, medicalized models of addiction, which may not align with everyone's experience or goals. These terms suggest a binary framework – either someone is "in recovery" (good) or has "relapsed" (bad) – which can lead to shame, self-blame, and discouragement if a person returns to drug use. Instead, using more neutral and person-centered language can reduce stigma. For example, instead of "recovery", phrases like "personal process", "growth journey", or "well-being path" acknowledge that change is nonlinear and individualized. Rather than "relapse", terms like "return to use", "setback", or "slip" recognize that substance use exists on a spectrum and that people can learn from their experiences without feeling like they've failed. By shifting language, we can foster compassionate, nonjudgmental conversations that empower people rather than shame them.

Drug policy and access to evidence-based care

Despite growing evidence supporting harm reduction approaches, most addiction treatment providers in the U.S. continue to prioritize abstinence-based models and do not integrate harm reduction into their services (Abraham et al., 2020; White, 2014). Many treatment programs remain influenced by traditional 12-step philosophies, which often reject harm reduction as enabling rather than recognizing its effectiveness in engaging individuals at various stages of change (Marlatt et al., 2012).

As authors committed to reshaping adolescent substance use care, we are regularly frustrated that – despite decades of data supporting buprenorphine – so few accessible, evidence-based options exist for youth, particularly for those who are low-income, uninsured, or part of marginalized communities. These gaps reflect the lasting imprint of drug war ideologies that prioritize abstinence and punishment over public health and equity. King et al.'s findings underscore how structural barriers and stigma continue to limit treatment access, disproportionately harming adolescents already burdened by systemic inequities.

Part II

Addressing Substance Use with Harm Reduction Treatment Strategies

Barry Lessin M.Ed., CAADC

The desire to alter consciousness is a natural and deeply human impulse—one that spans cultures, histories, and developmental stages. Andrew Weil (1973) and Norman Zinberg (1986) helped reframe this drive as normal rather than pathological, with Zinberg's *Drug, Set, and Setting* model highlighting how substance use is shaped by mindset, environment, and context—not just the drug itself. These foundational ideas paved the way for harm reduction approaches that challenge abstinence-only models and embrace a more compassionate, client-centered framework. This section traces the evolution of harm reduction psychotherapy through the work of pioneers like Marlatt, Denning, Little, Tatarsky, Springer, and Kellogg, while introducing core clinical tools that help therapists support change without judgment. In his groundbreaking book, *The Natural Mind*, Andrew Weil (2004) acknowledges that the desire to alter consciousness is a fundamental and natural part of the human experience. He recognized early on how damaging drug policies can be when he argued that seeking altered states of consciousness, whether through meditation, fasting, or drug use, is not inherently pathological but rather a natural inclination. He suggests that the problem lies not in the pursuit of these states but in the societal approach to drug use, which often criminalizes and stigmatizes it rather than understanding its roots in human nature.

We have thrived as a species by having our brains hard-wired to move toward pleasure and away from pain. People use substances for reasons (Tatarsky, 2003). Substances help us relax, sleep, have fun, improve creativity, and cope with the pain associated with more serious mental health issues. Within this framework, addictions can be viewed as compulsive behaviors gone awry (Stout, 2009, p. 45) driven by desires that pressure people to make choices about whether to participate in risky behavior; or use substances, as well as sex, food, gambling, and internet activity in potentially destructive ways. The compulsions are related to underlying psychological processes involving an interaction of psychosocial and emotional factors unique to each person.

While harm reduction has been the underlying paradigm for the interventions described above, it also influenced substance use treatment protocols. At the turn of the 21st century, a group of like-minded practitioners and researchers were increasingly frustrated with the lack of success with their substance using clients and started questioning the efficacy of the traditional models of substance use disorder (SUD) treatment they were working within. They began to develop ideas on how to integrate harm reduction concepts into a new approach to therapy. (Reminder, for the sake of consistency, we will use the term "traditional treatment" to refer to one-size-fits-all, abstinence-only models.)

The seminal work of harm reductionists Alan Marlatt (1996), William Miller (1991), Patt Denning and Jeannie Little (2012), and Andrew Tatarsky (2003) laid the foundation for a paradigm shift in addiction treatment. Together, they helped move the field away from rigid, patriarchal, and prescriptive models toward a more client-centered, collaborative, and nonjudgmental approach. This shift not only lowered barriers to care but also integrated a range of evidence-based therapies – including Cognitive Behavioral Therapy (CBT) (American Psychological Association, n.d.), Motivational Interviewing (MI) (Miller & Rollnick, 2012), and Dialectical Behavior Therapy (DBT) (Linehan, 2015) – into flexible, harm reduction–oriented frameworks.

Co-authors Pat Denning and Jeannie Little, as well as Andrew Tatarsky wrote books articulating their model for therapy that have become ad hoc training resources of interested therapists for the past several decades. A fundamental aspect of both Denning's and Tatarsky's therapy is to acknowledge that treatment is based on the *client's* needs and goals and that *any* change to reduce harms associated with substance use is important. Denning empowers clients by directly collaborating with them as "therapeutic teams", supporting them for positive change on their own terms (Denning & Little, 2012).

Tatarsky's model of Integrative Harm Reduction Psychotherapy emphasizes the integration of strategic skills-building, exploration of the multiple meanings of substance use, and the importance of the therapeutic alliance (Tatarsky, 2003). Scott Kellogg and Andrew Tatarsky (2012) outlined key measures to enhance clinical work with addiction: treating addiction within a psychiatric framework, prioritizing a strong therapeutic alliance, understanding patients through multi-faceted internal models, incorporating contingency management and positive reinforcement, viewing long-term healing through identity theory, and integrating recovery culture with formal treatment. Kellogg (2024) further emphasizes that adopting a harm reduction mindset allows therapists to be more relaxed, relinquish the need to dictate what's best for clients, and simply "love their clients".

We view harm reduction approaches to treatment as a needed alternative to the traditional treatment model. Unfortunately, the traditional treatment industry has been resistant to even exploring a shift in its approach. Additionally, the powerful and deeply ingrained stigma – rooted in drug policies shaped by War on Drugs narratives – continues to be a major barrier. As a result, comprehensive harm reduction services, including therapy, have struggled to gain wider acceptance as a legitimate practice. The gap that exists between the accessibility of harm reduction services and the need for them contributes to the millions of individuals and families remaining vulnerable to the harmful consequences of substance use (Vakharia, 2024).

Harm Reduction De-Stigmatizes Substance Use

A nonjudgmental, stigma-free approach to understanding the impact of a person's substance use is to contextualize a person's use as having a specific *relationship* with a substance or substances. It shifts away from substance demonization toward understanding the full context of use. Mid-century psychiatrist Norman Zinberg's pioneering Drug, Set, and Setting expectations research (Zinberg, 1986) is foundational in helping us understand the value of how all substance use can be understood within the context of a "relationship" with them. Relationships with substances are similar to our relationships with people – there are reasons for being in a relationship; there are benefits and drawbacks to being in any relationship; there is a relationship history, including ups and downs, a beginning, middle, and end. This approach reduces defensiveness and increases clients' motivation to explore their use, understanding that the substances they use are not the problem per se, but their relationship with them can be, as can be their relationship with people.

We will explore Drug, Set, and Setting in depth in Chapter 10, focusing on its clinical applications. For now, it is enough to understand that the drug (substance type and use patterns), set (individual mindset, expectations, and mental state), and setting (environmental and social context) interact to shape a person's substance use experience:

- Drug – What substances are used, in what quantities, and how frequently?
- Set (Mindset) – What internal factors (e.g., mood, expectations, mental health) influence use?
- Setting – In what environments does use occur? With whom? What risks and protective factors exist?

Viewed through this de-stigmatizing lens, people are better able to understand where the harms lie in their use and may be more likely to be motivated to explore their use and willing to take steps to make a change in their use. Also, when parents can embrace this relationship perspective, they tend to feel less anxious and more hopeful and empowered when having conversations with their teens about substances.

Even if change is desired, the process of change is frightening and it can sometimes feel overwhelming. Most people tend to resist changing all at once, and research shows that change occurs in predictable stages. This process is formally known as The Transtheoretical Model, or Stages of Change (SOC) model (discussed more fully in Chapter 10) and describes how change is not a single event, but a process, and individuals may fluctuate between stages before achieving lasting change. Understanding which stage someone is in can help tailor interventions to meet people where they are at and support their current needs. Family problems take some time to develop and will take some time to resolve.

Chapter 6

Key Considerations in Practicing HRT

Practicing Harm Reduction Therapy (HRT) requires more than adopting a new set of techniques; it involves a fundamental shift in how clinicians understand change, ethics, and the therapeutic relationship. For many providers trained in abstinence-based or pathology-focused models, this shift often begins with discomfort: recognizing that conventional tools may fall short – or even cause harm – when working with clients who aren't ready or able to pursue abstinence. The following section outlines key clinical considerations that emerge in the practice of HRT, including flexibility, neutrality, ethical engagement, and the dialectical stance required to navigate complexity. These principles are not abstract ideals – they reflect the lived challenges and growth of clinicians who have chosen to meet clients where they are, while still holding a deep commitment to safety, integrity, and therapeutic impact.

Harm reduction providers like us who began careers trained in traditional treatment models eventually bumped into conflicts that made it challenging – and often increased the likelihood of harm – to work with people motivated for change but didn't have the resources or support to engage in the abstinence-only model. Our attempts to engage them in treatment was a dilemma that created much discomfort because we found ourselves working within an ethical "gray" area, requiring us to go outside the limited traditional "allowable" toolkit of interventions. We realized that to maintain our ethical standards and continue using evidence-based treatments, we would need to make significant changes in how we viewed our clients and ourselves as therapists.

Denning and Little's discussion of this in *Practicing Harm Reduction Psychotherapy* (2012) resonated for us in addressing the challenge of providing harm reduction-based care because it was congruent with our experiences of being concerned about our responsibility for client care and not wanting to abandon them and their potential risky behavior. This dilemma implores us to embrace a core value of the Hippocratic Oath, "First Do No Harm". This is more than a passive guideline; it actively informs how we approach clients, emphasizing respect, collaboration, and safety. It ensures that therapeutic interventions support clients' well-being without adding to their challenges, focusing on reducing harm in both the therapeutic relationship and the broader context of their lives (Denning & Little, 2012, p. 3).

Harm reduction, at its core, is grounded in a person-centered philosophy, making it a natural fit for many therapists trained in the foundational concepts of Abraham Maslow's Humanistic Psychology (1970) and Carl Rogers' Person-Centered Therapy (1961). Person-Centered Therapy emphasizes the client's autonomy, perspective, and innate capacity for growth, aligning seamlessly with harm reduction principles. Both approaches center on forming a collaborative partnership in which the client's self-determination is honored, and their lived experience is recognized as a vital source of insight in the therapeutic process. This approach fosters a dynamic relationship rooted in mutual respect and trust.

While we describe our work as "person-centered", Denning and Little (2012, pp. 293–294) bring to light the subconscious realities of our nature as human beings to get a truer sense of what is specifically required in working most effectively with substance users. Practicing true person-centeredness becomes particularly complex when working with individuals who may be at risk themselves or pose risks to others, as it requires balancing empathy and support with careful consideration of safety and accountability.

Infinite Flexibility

Expanding on the limitations of just being person-centered, Denning and Little (2012) describe the concept of being "infinitely flexible" (p. 293). Flexibility in this context goes beyond being merely eclectic. It refers to the ability of a therapist to adjust their approach, techniques, and interventions according to the specific needs and context of the client, sometimes pivoting at a moment's notice. It emphasizes the therapist's capacity to "meet the client where they are", adapting in real-time to the client's situation, behavior, and readiness for change. This could involve switching between different therapeutic techniques, theories, or interventions based on what is most useful for the client *at that moment*.

The implications of infinite flexibility are that the therapist is prepared to abandon their usual stance, training, or preconceived notions to align with the client's current needs, whether that means being more directive or more passive, more structured or more open. As we evolve as therapists, we develop a therapeutic orientation which ultimately reflects *our* worldview, not that of the client. Harm reduction is a *comprehensive worldview*, not simply a technique or theory of behavior. And because this worldview inherently includes our personal narratives, values and judgments, it's crucial to recognize how these biases can inadvertently interfere with our ability to connect authentically with clients. This means embracing the client's perspective and remaining open to all outcomes without imposing our beliefs or predetermined theories. The therapist's role is not to impose judgment or enforce rules but to partner with the client in their journey toward health, however, that may manifest. This is especially important in situations where the client may resist traditional therapeutic methods due to their previous negative experiences with therapy (Denning & Little, 2012, p. 293).

Denning and Little analogize this to the business adage, "the customer is always right". Harm reduction therapists recognize that when clients challenge us, our ability to truly listen hinges on letting them feel "right" in the moment. This sense of validation fosters a sense of safety that allows clients to engage more deeply in the therapeutic process, especially when addressing areas of tension or difference.

This therapeutic flexibility is particularly important when working with clients who may have multiple diagnoses or complex needs. Therapists want to be trained to handle these complexities while also learning to step back and allow clients to lead the direction of therapy. Effective HRT demands that therapists hold a space for clients to express themselves, explore their behaviors, and make decisions about their own treatment.

Radical Neutrality

Intertwined with infinite flexibility, Denning and Little (2012) emphasize that effective harm reduction therapists are able to practice "radical neutrality". Originally drawing on ideas from systemic family therapy (Bowen, 1978) and classical psychoanalysis (Greenson, 1967), radical neutrality suggests that therapists maintain a stance of non-alignment and intense curiosity.

In practice, this means neither condemning nor endorsing the client's substance use; instead, it is being a witness to the client's vulnerability and allowing the client to feel fully heard, free from your personal agendas or preconceived judgments. While it might feel counterintuitive by not "guiding" or "advising", especially when risky behavior is shared, radical neutrality trusts that clients, when truly heard, can uncover insights and take ownership of their choices. You remain open to exploring every angle: What functions does substance use serve? In what ways has it been helpful or harmful? Could there be intermediate steps – like using less frequently, trying safer methods, or building a supportive network – to reduce immediate risks?

The *righting reflex* is a concept from Motivational Interviewing (MI), developed by William R. Miller and Stephen Rollnick. It refers to the natural tendency of people – especially helpers, counselors, and professionals – to try to immediately "fix" a person's problem by offering advice, solutions, or corrections. While well-meaning, the righting reflex can often backfire, especially when working with people who are ambivalent about change (Miller & Rollnick, 2012).

It's natural for therapists to initially wrestle with doubts of condoning dangerous behaviors by staying neutral. However, radical neutrality doesn't mean ignoring ethical or safety concerns. It means offering harm reduction tools like safer use strategies, overdose prevention education, and other risk-reduction methods without imposing a moral verdict on the client's lifestyle. This blended approach of harm reduction psychotherapy and radical neutrality can be especially powerful for clients who have felt shamed, rejected, or traumatized by previous treatment experiences. Our clients have expressed profound appreciation for finding HRT after having negative traditional treatment experiences. Our adolescent clients realize that treatment is not akin to what feels like, to them, detention with their disciplinarian vice principal in school.

The traditional model left us with few options when our clients were not successful meeting the expected goal of abstinence. It was liberating for us as therapists when, as harm reduction therapists, we began to collaborate with clients on goals or behavior changes they deemed important. An epiphany in our experiences transitioning to harm reduction occurred when we encountered the adage: "when your only tool is a hammer every problem appears to be a nail".

Rather than pressuring them to conform to a single vision of recovery, you show that you value their autonomy and trust their capacity for growth. By maintaining curiosity about their lived experiences – and allowing them to define success on their own terms – you foster a therapeutic alliance built on respect and authenticity. It demands from us a deep dedication to introspection, self-awareness, and personal growth. And the need to know when to, and be willing to, get out of the way of the client.

MI, which we explore further in Chapter 10, embraces radical neutrality by emphasizing collaboration, and evocation, or facilitating the client's self-discovery of motivations for change, rather than imposing external directives, as the therapist remains open and curious about the client's experience without trying to steer them toward a specific path. MI's focus on acknowledging ambivalence and respecting the client's autonomy allows therapists to offer support while respecting the client's personal decision-making process.

The Dialectical Nature of Harm Reduction Psychotherapy

Denning and Little describe a dialectical aspect of harm reduction psychotherapy – one that holds multiple, seemingly opposing, truths or strategies at the same time. Clinicians must be highly trained and experienced to navigate clients with complex, co-occurring conditions, are actively using drugs, and facing significant health and safety risks while simultaneously being willing to "know nothing". This "knowing nothing" involves fully joining with the client, setting aside preconceived notions and expertise, and meeting them exactly where they are in their journey (Denning & Little, 2012, p. 294).

This dual capacity – to bring expertise and humility together – lies in the heart of HRT. It requires a level of skill and confidence that comes from experiencing success with moving clients towards their treatment goals enabling us to let go of the mantle of expert. Appreciating that our clients know themselves best and that we can learn a lot from our clients by giving them this space helps us gain confidence and the courage needed to let go of our previous roles of "authority" and "expert", allowing clients to have the agency to tell their own lived experience.

Supervision and Training

Individual and group supervision are crucial components of a harm reduction therapist's experience, providing a structured space to navigate complex clinical, ethical, and legal issues. Topics such as assessing suicidal or homicidal risk, mandatory reporting of child and elder abuse, and maintaining professional boundaries in dual relationships are often outlined in clinical policy manuals, yet require active discussion, case-based learning, and experiential exercises such as role-playing and clinical vignettes to enhance comprehension and application. Harm reduction providers working with dually diagnosed clients frequently encounter emotionally intense and ethically challenging situations that cannot be fully addressed in policy and procedure manuals of employers (Denning & Little, 2012).

Supervision plays an additional role in fostering reflective practice, where clinicians can explore ethical dilemmas, process case-specific challenges, and maintain alignment with harm reduction principles. Engaging in this self-reflective and discussion-based process enables therapists to recognize and manage personal biases, countertransference, and navigate difficult emotions.

In addition to supervision, ongoing training opportunities (National Harm Reduction Coalition, n.d.) are essential to keep clinicians informed about the latest knowledge and best practices and contribute to developing the confidence and competence necessary for real-world application. Staying updated on the pharmacology of alcohol and emerging drugs is crucial, especially as new, or "novel", substances appear on the streets (Vakharia & Little, 2017).

The Challenge of Establishing Empirical Support for HRT

HRT has gained recognition as a compassionate and practical alternative to abstinence-based treatment, yet it faces persistent challenges in establishing empirical support within traditional research frameworks. Unlike rigid treatment models that emphasize complete abstinence as the primary outcome, HRT is flexible, individualized, and focused on reducing harm rather than enforcing total sobriety. This variability, while beneficial for client-centered care, creates difficulties in designing standardized, controlled studies that fit conventional evidence-based treatment (EBT) criteria (Denning & Little, 2012).

A primary issue in measuring the effectiveness of HRT is the lack of a singular, uniform outcome measure. Traditional substance use treatment research often evaluates success through binary outcomes, such as whether an individual remains abstinent for a specified period.

HRT, however, values incremental progress, safer use, improved well-being, and enhanced quality of life, all of which are difficult to quantify in standardized trials (Tatarsky, 2002). This challenge is compounded by the fact that clients set their own goals, which vary widely, ranging from reducing frequency of use to using in safer environments or even continuing use with greater self-awareness. The absence of rigid endpoints makes it harder to apply randomized controlled trial (RCT) methodologies, which favor interventions with clear, predefined outcomes.

Another barrier to empirical validation is that HRT operates in real-world, community-based settings, rather than controlled laboratory environments. Research models that prioritize RCTs struggle to accommodate the complexities of harm reduction interventions, which often involve multiple components, individualized treatment plans, and a high degree of therapist adaptability (Vakharia & Little, 2017). Unlike abstinence-based programs, which offer structured, time-limited treatment protocols, HRT encourages ongoing engagement without predefined termination points, making it difficult to track long-term outcomes through traditional research designs. Furthermore, ethical concerns about randomly assigning individuals to abstinence-only or harm reduction conditions create obstacles in generating comparative data.

Scott Kellogg (2013) also highlights the institutional resistance to harm reduction research, noting that funding bodies, regulatory agencies, and mainstream treatment organizations have historically favored abstinence-based approaches. Many grant providers and academic institutions hesitate to support studies that do not frame abstinence as the ultimate goal, leading to a shortage of large-scale, well-funded research on harm reduction therapy. Additionally, researchers face challenges in securing approval from institutional review boards (IRBs), as harm reduction strategies – such as supervised drug use or maintenance therapies – are sometimes misinterpreted as enabling substance use rather than providing a pathway for risk reduction.

Despite these challenges, harm reduction therapy has amassed strong practice-based evidence through clinical case studies, qualitative research, and community-driven data. Denning, Tatarsky, Vakharia, and Kellogg advocate for more flexible research models that prioritize client-centered outcomes, real-world effectiveness, and longitudinal engagement over rigid abstinence-based metrics. As harm reduction continues to gain global recognition as a public health approach, the challenge remains to develop research methodologies that capture its complexity while maintaining scientific rigor. Moving forward, the integration of qualitative, mixed-methods, and participatory action research may provide a more accurate reflection of HRT's effectiveness, allowing it to gain broader acceptance within the evidence-based treatment landscape.

Chapter 7

Core Dilemmas in Practicing Harm Reduction Therapy

Core Dilemmas in Practicing Harm Reduction Therapy

Harm Reduction Therapy (HRT) challenges clinicians to navigate a range of ethical, clinical, and relational tensions that do not always arise in traditional treatment models. This section explores several core dilemmas that are inherent to practicing HRT, particularly with adolescents. Drawing on the work of Denning and Little (2012), we examine how therapists must often balance opposing forces such as structure and flexibility, neutrality and engagement, and safety and autonomy. Rather than offering fixed solutions, these dilemmas call for ongoing self-reflection, clinical humility, and a commitment to client-centered practice. Each of the following subsections introduces one of these core tensions, illustrated by clinical examples and practical considerations for integrating harm reduction principles.

Balancing process and content

The tension between following structured assessment protocols and allowing space for client-driven exploration is a central concern in harm reduction therapy. Therapists must gather essential information about substance use and risk without overwhelming clients with rigid procedures. The aim is to balance safety with engagement from the very start. The following section takes a closer look at how harm reduction therapists approach assessment as an ongoing, collaborative process rather than a one-time intake task.

Many programs require formal, systematic intake assessments before treatment begins with the goals of accurately diagnosing conditions and identifying co-occurring disorders, urgent needs, and risk factors. Traditional psychotherapy often prioritizes process over content, allowing the client to set the focus of discussions rather than systematically assessing their daily experiences. However, in HRT, direct questioning and attention to detail are crucial, especially regarding substance use and other risky behaviors. The challenge is to intuit how to balance structured assessment with a client-driven approach, ensuring that clients are not burdened by rigid intake procedures while still gathering important information.

Example: Fifteen-year-old Liz was caught smoking cannabis in school and was required to seek a substance use evaluation as a condition for returning to school. In the initial intake session, worried about possible sanctions from the school, Liz is overwhelmed by specific questions about her substance use patterns and mental health concerns. Recognizing this, the counselor, Jean, needs to adjust her approach, asking only the most essential questions to ensure Liz's immediate safety – such as the current amount and frequency of cannabis use levels and any potential harmful consequences – while allowing the client to share her story in her own words. In subsequent sessions, Jean gently revisits necessary topics like mental health and support systems, ensuring that critical information is gathered over time. This approach balances the process (client-centered conversations) with the necessary content (comprehensive assessment), making Liz feel heard and respected while ensuring that vital clinical information is obtained for effective support.

We identify the importance of the balance between process and content further when we review the Integrated Dynamic Engagement Assessment (IDEA) in Chapter 10.

Initiating versus responding

The clinical tension between taking a proactive stance and following the client's lead is a common dynamic in harm reduction therapy. Therapists often adjust their style based on the client's level of engagement, risk factors, and developmental readiness. What follows is an exploration of how harm reduction practitioners navigate this flexibility while staying grounded in client-centered values.

Therapists must continuously adjust their approach to maintain trust while providing essential interventions. Some therapists may struggle with the active engagement required in HRT, such as investigating drug use patterns, providing education, or teaching harm-reduction skills. While some clinicians prefer a passive, insight-oriented approach, HRT often necessitates active interventions to assess risk and introduce harm-reducing strategies. Therapists must be aware of each client's tolerance for engagement; some may need a highly interactive approach, while others may feel overwhelmed by therapist-led discussions.

Example: A therapist, Ben, is working with a high school senior, Sam, who was referred by his parents after they discovered that he was misusing prescribed opiates after his orthopedic surgery. He expressed little concern about his use, and initially, Ben takes a responsive Motivational Interviewing (MI) approach, listening to Sam's experiences and allowing him to guide the conversation. However, when Sam mentions that he is having difficulty tapering his use, Ben recognizes the need for more active engagement and shifts to an initiating stance, asking direct but non-judgmental questions about possible physical dependence and provides information on opiate dependence and withdrawal. At the same time, Ben remains attuned to Sam's comfort level, ensuring the conversation doesn't feel intrusive. This balance helps Sam feel supported while also receiving critical information to reduce potential harm. We identify how MI provides a framework for managing the initiating versus responding dynamic in Chapter 10.

Depth versus behavioral focus

Integrating behavioral risk-reduction strategies with deeper psychological work is a core task in HRT. The next section explores how therapists can hold both aims – reducing immediate harm while addressing underlying emotional, relational, or developmental issues – in a cohesive and responsive clinical approach.

Substance use can become self-perpetuating, requiring concrete behavioral tools alongside insight-based therapy. The challenge lies in supporting behavioral change without disrupting the therapeutic relationship or reinforcing stigma. Traditional psychodynamic and humanistic therapies often prioritize long-term insight development, assuming that resolving emotional conflicts will naturally lead to behavioral change. However, when substance dependence reaches a certain level, it can develop a "life of its own", becoming self-sustaining and operating independently of initial intentions. It is then that addressing the underlying psychological issues alone is insufficient. What often happens here is that the therapist will refer their client to an "addiction specialist", or even more disruptively, to a higher level of care such as an intensive outpatient program or inpatient rehab. The expectation is that the substance use will be addressed separately and once that is addressed, the client will return to the original therapist.

The authors have experienced this scenario many times, and this approach is effective when there is collaboration between the providers and a few precautions are taken. The primary therapist needs to be sensitive to the possibility that a referral to another therapist for their client's substance use, even temporarily, can feel stigmatizing and traumatizing to the client, especially if the client has abandonment issues. A frequent knee-jerk reaction by referring therapists is to immediately suggest residential rehab when a client's substance use becomes a concern. While well-intended, this approach often overlooks the fact that residential treatment is rarely necessary and may not be the best fit for the client's needs. Of course, if the client's substance use and/or risky behavior is becoming unstable, they may benefit from the structure of an intensive outpatient program or the stability provided by residential care. However, rather than assuming a higher level of care is required, the existing therapeutic relationship can be a powerful asset in supporting change. The referring therapist holds unique insight and trust with the client, making them well-positioned to integrate harm reduction strategies into treatment. This moment presents an opportunity for collaboration, education, and reinforcing that effective substance use treatment does not always require separation from the primary therapist. By embracing harm reduction principles, therapists can expand their skill set and better support clients without unnecessary disruption to care.

Example: Katy, a 16-year-old, has been experimenting with alcohol and cannabis, often using them to cope with stress from school and family conflicts. Her therapist, Susan, initially focused on exploring Katy's emotional struggles, aiming to build insight into how these stressors contribute to substance use. However, Susan realizes that Katy's substance use has become more frequent and poses immediate risks, requiring more direct intervention. To provide Katy with specialized support, Susan refers her to a harm reduction specialist who educates her about her "relationship with substances" and offers practical strategies to reduce substance-related harm. While Susan continues working on Katy's emotional challenges, the harm reduction specialist focuses on concrete behavioral changes. This collaborative approach ensures Katy receives both immediate support for her substance use and deeper therapeutic care, helping her feel supported on multiple levels.

By integrating behavioral interventions with deeper therapeutic work, harm reduction therapists avoid further stigmatizing or traumatizing the client. The impact on clients is significant: they feel understood and cared for, knowing that their emotional well-being is being addressed while also receiving practical tools to stay safe. This balanced approach helps them trust the therapeutic process and feel empowered to make healthier choices without feeling judged or overwhelmed.

Therapeutic neutrality and engagement

This section revisits the challenge of maintaining therapeutic neutrality, while deeply engaging with clients who may need care outside conventional settings. Therapists may need to offer expanded accessibility and flexibility, all while remaining grounded in ethical, intentional practice.

We introduced the idea of radical neutrality as one of the challenges of HRT in Chapter 6, and it requires us to step beyond our comfort zone to balance the clinical tension of applying therapeutic neutrality to effectively engage with our clients. Examples of this are when HRT may need to extend beyond the traditional therapy setting, such as offering phone check-ins during high-risk times (e.g., "cocktail hour"), meeting clients in public or community spaces for sessions, or conducting home visits for medically fragile clients. These are operational examples of "meeting clients where they are", fostering trust and reducing barriers to care.

Ethical Considerations in Harm Reduction

An ethical framework rooted in client autonomy, nonmaleficence (doing no harm), and social justice underpins HRT. Because HRT departs from abstinence-only models, therapists are often called to navigate complex moral and legal dilemmas while staying aligned with harm reduction values. The following discussion examines how this ethical foundation shapes real-world clinical decision-making.

Ethics in counseling and psychotherapy encompasses the adherence to moral principles and is based on the principles of justice, fairness, honesty, integrity, and respect. These promote good and avoid harm, contributing positively to the well-being of individuals or society and avoiding unnecessary suffering. Different professions have their own ethical codes, which set the standard for appropriate conduct. Similarly, communities or cultures may have shared moral values that define what is considered ethical behavior. Ethics include responsible and accountable behavior that involves taking responsibility for one's actions and being accountable for the consequences of those actions.

Because harm reduction is an oft-contested break from traditional addiction treatment, it is imperative to pay close attention to its ethical underpinnings (Denning & Little, 2012, p. 297). We are all taught ethics as part of our professional training and are required to have a command of the principles in order to pass licensing exams, but the theoretical foundation of ethics in HRT is infrequently taught. Since harm reduction is grounded in the belief that people should have the right to make choices about their own health, even when those choices involve behaviors typically seen as harmful, ethical considerations revolve around the principle of nonmaleficence and beneficence (doing good).

The ethical debate surrounding harm reduction can be controversial, especially in relation to issues like overdose prevention facilities or the right to self-medicate. Some argue that drug use, like any other form of personal behavior, should not be criminalized if it does not harm others. They believe in protecting individuals' rights to make personal decisions about their health and bodies. Others may feel that addiction compromises an individual's autonomy, making it justifiable to intervene in their decision-making. These are the kinds of ethical issues that harm reduction therapists must navigate as they support their clients in managing their health and behavior.

Ethical dilemmas may arise when therapists feel torn between their duty to the client and the broader societal pressures that might prioritize public health and safety. For example, should a therapist support a client's decision to engage in risky behaviors if it aligns with the client's personal choices? HRT advocates for the recognition of these complex ethical issues and encourages therapists to practice with compassion, understanding that clients may need time to make changes, and that even small steps toward improvement are significant.

Radical neutrality presents an ethical dilemma by requiring therapists to suspend judgment while still acknowledging potential harm. Philosopher and ethicist John Kleinig (2008) argues that true neutrality isn't possible, since our assessment of what constitutes harm is inherently subjective. While neutrality is important for creating a non-judgmental therapeutic space, it often demands a moral compromise – therapists must take a stand, even as they strive to respect autonomy. Kleinig warns that complete neutrality can lead to moral neglect if it prevents us from confronting the real consequences of risky behavior. The challenge is to maintain a neutral stance without ignoring the moral implications when clients engage in behaviors that may cause serious harm (Denning & Little, 2012, p. 301).

Demanding inclusion of people who use drugs (PWUD) in treatment programming

Emphasizing the importance of involving people with lived experience in shaping the systems meant to serve them, the upcoming discussion draws on values of self-determination, equity, and accountability, while also recognizing that meaningful inclusion requires ethical consideration and clear structure.

Building on the discussion from Chapter 1 about involving people who use drugs (PWUD) in shaping the services intended for them, it is worth acknowledging a slogan from the disability rights movement: "Nothing About Us Without Us." This phrase highlights a core harm reduction value that people with lived experience must be meaningfully included in decisions that affect their lives – not as passive recipients, but as active participants in designing, implementing, and evaluating services. Especially treatment centers. When a new facility is proposed, the loudest voices are local businesses and homeowners, not the people who desperately need access to care. Decisions are made based on property values and public safety fears, not on whether the center is actually accessible for those relying on public transportation. Meanwhile, clients are expected to navigate rigid schedules, impossible intake hours, and endless red tape, as if these barriers aren't the very things keeping them from getting help. The real experts – the ones who know the struggles, limitations, and solutions firsthand – are left out of the process entirely. The harm reduction community insists that the people most affected by these policies deserve a seat at the table, because they know best what they need (Vakharia, 2017).

However, simply including people with lived experience in decision-making is not enough; how they are engaged matters just as much as whether they are included. While harm reduction emphasizes the importance of peer-led interventions, poorly designed or unsupported engagement efforts can have unintended consequences, particularly for at-risk youth. Paterson and Panessa (2008) caution that without adequate structure and support, peer-led initiatives can unintentionally reinforce harmful behaviors or normalize risky substance use. They emphasize that poorly implemented engagement strategies – especially those involving at-risk youth – may lead to unintended negative consequences, including the promotion of harmful norms.

Ethical themes in harm reduction

Key ethical issues – such as autonomy versus paternalism, informed consent, stigma, and resource allocation – will be examined next, offering a framework for navigating the ethical complexity often encountered in harm reduction practice.

Autonomy versus Paternalism: One of the core ethical debates in HRT revolves around autonomy: the client's right to make their own choices, and paternalism: where a therapist might feel a responsibility to act in the client's best interest, even against their wishes. HRT places a strong emphasis on client autonomy, encouraging individuals to make their own decisions about behavior change. This raises the ethical question of how much control a therapist should give the client, especially when the client's behavior can be harmful to their health or safety. On the other hand, since in many cultures, abstinence from substances is often seen as a demonstration of personal discipline and respect for both oneself and the community, some clinicians may feel a moral obligation to intervene or push for abstinence, even if it goes against the client's wishes. The ethical dilemma here is determining when it is appropriate to override a client's autonomy to ensure their safety or well-being (e.g., in the case of suicidal ideation or overdose risk). Critics argue that harm reduction may enable certain behaviors by accepting them as a normal part of life and therefore undermining the moral goal of complete abstinence. This issue hinges on whether the goal of therapy should focus on reducing harm and improving quality of life – even if this means accepting some degree of risk – or whether total abstinence from harmful behaviors is a more ethical goal.

Informed Consent: Informed consent is a critical ethical issue because therapists need to make sure clients are fully aware of the risks associated with their behaviors, as well as the potential outcomes of harm reduction strategies, such as safer drug use or non-abstinence-focused approaches. Are clients receiving adequate information about the risks involved in harm reduction strategies (e.g., the continued use of drugs even in reduced amounts)? Can clients truly make informed decisions about their care when the therapy itself may not aim for total cessation of risky behaviors? The challenge for the therapist is to carefully navigate the ethical duty to ensure that the client understands the full scope of potential risks while respecting their right to make their own decisions about their health and behavior.

Stigma: The stigma of substance use is a persistent issue in ethics in HRT. Substance users often face significant social stigma, which can interfere with their access to care, their self-esteem, and their willingness to engage in treatment. It's imperative that harm reduction therapists actively acknowledge and confront the broader societal context in which clients' behaviors are judged and stigmatized, and continuously engage in self-reflection to mitigate biases and avoid contributing to the marginalization of clients. The author's experience with ingrained stigma took years to shake after his practice shifted to a harm reduction approach, and he still catches himself confronting unwitting biases. This raises the question of whether therapists can ever be fully free from their own implicit biases. Recognizing and addressing these biases is an ongoing process, requiring humility, education, and a commitment to truly seeing clients beyond the moral and social judgments imposed on them.

Resource Allocation and Access to Care: Access to harm reduction services is often limited by socioeconomic factors, geographical location, and healthcare policies. For instance, in many regions, there are insufficient resources and support for providing harm reduction services, such as overdose prevention centers or needle exchange programs. Should harm reduction services be considered a universal right or a specialized treatment? What is the ethical responsibility of healthcare systems to provide equitable access to harm reduction services, particularly for marginalized populations, including people who inject drugs or those in lower-income communities? There are also ethical challenges related to funding and political support for harm reduction strategies. Should resources be diverted from abstinence-focused programs to those that support harm reduction, particularly when there may be a lack of political will to support these initiatives?

Ethics and Mandated Treatment

Exploring how therapists can ethically support clients within mandated care systems while minimizing harm and preserving autonomy, the following discussion considers the conflict between coercive frameworks and harm reduction values, offering alternative strategies for engagement.

Mandated substance use treatment is used by courts, employers, families, and child protective services but HRT is incompatible with coerced treatment. Criminal justice and child protective system mandates often reflect punitive approaches rooted in the War on Drugs. Detaining individuals in the name of drug treatment frequently occurs in settings that fail to provide appropriate treatment and can serve as venues for abuse. Decisions to use mandated treatment may be driven less by evidence than by ideology, stigma, and limited access to voluntary treatment (Bazazi, 2018).

The assumption that all drug use is harmful ignores the complexities of individual experiences, including cases where people manage trauma more effectively with substance use. Supporters of mandated substance use treatment compare it to life-saving medical interventions, but this is a misleading analogy as it ignores the complexities of addiction and autonomy in treatment and it assumes mandated treatment is as effective and ethically sound as urgent medical intervention. Unlike a medical emergency where a patient cannot refuse treatment, HRT recognizes that clients have enough agency to opt out of treatment. Also, while the intent of mandated treatment is often to reduce harm and promote health, it can paradoxically lead to adverse outcomes, such as increased risk of overdose post-treatment, which arises because individuals may lose tolerance during enforced abstinence, making them more susceptible to overdose upon a using slip (Wild et al., 2018).

Families impacted by hazardous substance use at times will become so exasperated by their loved one's ongoing risky behaviors harming themselves and putting their families at risk, that they feel compelled to take action to coerce their loved one into getting help. These family mandates differ from societal or medical mandates because close relationships – such as family, friends, teachers, and colleagues – are personally or professionally affected by a drug user's behavior. These individuals have both the right to protect themselves and a degree of responsibility to support the safety and well-being of the user, depending on their relationship and the user's age. Similarly, communities have a vested interest in addressing substance use among their members. Some argue that the criminal justice system serves to protect society from the harms of drug use. However, this perception is flawed for two main reasons: drug use, though criminalized, is often a victimless crime, and drug laws are disproportionately enforced against people of color. This raises the question of whether these communities are being targeted out of genuine concern or for other, less justifiable reasons.

Ethical Engagement in Mandated Care

Building on these ideas, harm reduction offers a valuable lens for navigating the complexities of treatment under external pressure or legal mandate. It introduces concepts like psychological reactance, clarifying why clients may resist even well-intentioned interventions, and, crucially, it equips therapists to maintain a collaborative stance despite external demands. The following section examines how harm reduction can support clinical decision-making in these contexts, balancing engagement and autonomy.

Balancing mandates with a client-centered, harm reduction approach is challenging. Traditional models rely on pressure to drive change, yet people often resist such directives, even when consequences are serious. This resistance, known as psychological reactance (Denning & Little, 2012, p. 38), underscores the value of approaches that build trust, support motivation, and promote self-directed change. Rather than relying on drug testing or punitive measures to enforce compliance, meeting clients where they are allows for a more effective therapeutic process. The Stages of Change (SOC) model discussed in Chapter 10 provides a framework for guiding this work, encouraging reflection on personal goals and challenging absolutes like "I don't have a choice" or "there's no other option". Exploring the reasoning behind these statements creates space for genuine, lasting change. When someone chooses to meet a mandate – such as maintaining sobriety to regain custody of a child – harm reduction strategies ensure that the process remains realistic and sustainable. Ultimately, harm reduction supports individuals in navigating their own realities rather than forcing conformity to a predetermined path (Denning & Little, 2012).

Balancing Ethical, Liability, Risk, and Legal Considerations

This section provides guidance on how to manage legal and ethical responsibilities – especially when working with adolescents. It discusses how to handle confidentiality, documentation, mandated reporting, and liability without sacrificing therapeutic trust.

HRT presents unique ethical, legal, and liability challenges, particularly when working with high-risk adolescents in harm reduction settings. Unlike abstinence-based models with clear-cut legal and ethical frameworks, harm reduction requires therapists to navigate a more nuanced landscape, balancing client autonomy with the duty to prevent harm. This demands careful attention to both clinical and relational aspects of treatment, as well as broader legal and professional responsibilities, including mandated reporting and liability mitigation. One of the central ethical dilemmas in adolescent HRT is balancing the minor's right to autonomy with parental and legal obligations. Adolescents are in a unique developmental stage where they are striving for independence, yet legally and ethically, they are often not granted full agency over their health decisions. Harm reduction therapists must navigate this tension of working within gray areas carefully, ensuring that interventions respect the adolescent's autonomy while adhering to legal and ethical mandates for safety and well-being.

A significant challenge is confidentiality; many adolescents will only engage in therapy if they feel safe discussing their substance use without fear of parental punishment or legal consequences. However, state laws vary regarding whether minors can consent to substance use treatment without parental involvement (English & Gudeman, 2024). Therapists must clearly explain confidentiality limitations to adolescent clients, ensuring they understand what can and cannot be kept private, especially when there is a risk of harm to themselves or others (Ford et al., 2023).

Therapists are legally required to report cases where an adolescent is at imminent risk of harm due to substance use, exploitation, or co-occurring concerns such as self-harm or abuse. However, defining what constitutes "imminent risk" in a harm reduction framework can be difficult. For example, should a therapist report a 16-year-old who regularly binge drinks but has no immediate health crisis? Or should intervention only occur if there is evidence of alcohol poisoning or endangerment?

A detailed case example in the sidebar illustrates the ethical and legal challenges explored, offering a practical lens on harm reduction with high-risk youth.

Case Example: Ethical and Legal Challenges in HRT with a High-Risk Adolescent

Client background:

Jake, a 16-year-old high school junior, was referred to therapy after being caught vaping cannabis at school, resulting in a two-week suspension. His parents, frustrated by his substance use, are pressuring him to enter an abstinence-based treatment program, believing it to be the best path forward. However, Jake does not see his vaping as a serious issue. He insists that it helps him manage stress and social anxiety, and he expresses reluctance to stop altogether. This dynamic creates a complex therapeutic landscape, requiring careful navigation of confidentiality, harm reduction planning, parental involvement, and legal liability.

Confidentiality versus parental Involvement:

While Jake is willing to discuss his substance use openly, he is adamant that his parents should not be involved in his treatment. This presents an immediate challenge, as minors' rights to confidentiality vary by state and often depend on the level of risk posed by their behavior. The therapist takes time to explain the legal limitations of confidentiality, ensuring that Jake understands what information can be kept private and what may need to be disclosed. By clarifying these boundaries early, the therapist builds trust and encourages honest discussions while ensuring compliance with state laws.

Mandated reporting and harm reduction planning:

During the therapy session, Jake shares that he sometimes drives after vaping, though he insists that he is "not too high" when doing so. This raises immediate ethical and safety concerns, as driving under the influence presents serious risks to himself and others. Instead of reacting with alarm or issuing ultimatums, the therapist uses Motivational Interviewing (MI), as outlined in Chapter 10, to help Jake reflect on his choices:

"On a scale of 1 to 10, how safe do you feel driving after vaping?"
"What's a situation where driving under the influence could go badly?"

Through this guided self-reflection, Jake acknowledges that his judgment may be impaired, even if he doesn't always notice it. Rather than resisting the conversation, he agrees to implement a harm reduction strategy – committing to a self-imposed rule not to drive within two hours of vaping. This approach honors Jake's autonomy while promoting a safer behavioral shift, reducing the immediate risks associated with his substance use.

Parental expectations versus adolescent autonomy:

Jake's parents, believing that any level of substance use is unacceptable, advocate for strict abstinence and insist on weekly drug testing as part of his treatment plan. The therapist, recognizing that forced abstinence often leads to secrecy and resistance, takes the time to educate the parents on harm reduction principles. They discuss how non-punitive, open communication can be more effective in reducing risky behavior than a strictly disciplinary approach.

As a result of these conversations, a compromise is reached: Jake agrees to reduce his vaping frequency and practice safer use (e.g., avoiding driving while high, limiting use to certain situations); and his parents agree to move away from punitive measures and instead focus on open dialogue and gradual behavior change. This negotiated approach supports Jake's autonomy while maintaining parental involvement, fostering a collaborative, trust-based environment rather than one built on control and surveillance.

Navigating liability concerns:

Given the ethical and legal complexities of Jake's case, the therapist ensures that comprehensive documentation is maintained throughout treatment, including: Jake's substance use patterns and his evolving understanding of the associated risks; the harm reduction strategies discussed, including his agreement to avoid driving within two hours of vaping; and justification for not reporting the case to child protective services, as Jake is engaging in risk reduction behaviors and does not appear to be in immediate danger. By thoroughly documenting these details, the therapist protects against liability, demonstrating a thoughtful, evidence-based approach that prioritizes client safety while respecting his autonomy.

Jake's case illustrates the complex balance that harm reduction therapists must strike when working with adolescents, where confidentiality, mandated reporting, parental involvement, and liability often intersect. A flexible, client-centered approach – integrating Motivational Interviewing (MI), harm reduction strategies, and parent education – can promote both safety and self-determination, allowing adolescents to make safer choices without alienation or resistance. This approach meets teens where they are and supports developmentally appropriate, ethical change.

Using MI and harm reduction techniques, addressed in more detail in Chapter 10, helps teens explore safer use without imposing abstinence, fostering collaboration over confrontation. This is especially effective for adolescents who don't view their use as problematic but are open to small, risk-reducing changes. Parental engagement within a harm reduction framework – rather than an abstinence-only mindset – can improve trust, communication, and outcomes. Educating caregivers shifts the focus from punishment to collaborative problem-solving. Finally, therapists must maintain thorough documentation of safety planning, harm reduction strategies, and reporting decisions to reduce liability and demonstrate ethical care (COSSUP, n.d.). Staying informed on minor consent laws and consulting legal professionals ensures therapists uphold their responsibilities while prioritizing adolescent autonomy and safety.

Cultural Responsiveness

Cultural responsiveness is not just an ethical imperative in adolescent harm reduction – it is foundational to building trust, relevance, and therapeutic alliance. The following section explores how culture shapes adolescents' experiences with substance use, identity, and healing, and offers strategies for providing care that honors the full complexity of their lived contexts.

Cultural responsiveness is fundamentally tied to ethical practice – especially in adolescent harm reduction – because it ensures that care is respectful, relevant, and grounded in the client's lived experience. Ethical principles such as autonomy, promoting well-being, avoiding harm, and ensuring fairness all depend on a clinician's ability to understand and honor the cultural frameworks that shape how adolescents view health, behavior, identity, and support. Cultural responsiveness is not optional in HRT – it is central to engagement, trust-building, and clinical relevance. Every adolescent brings a complex web of cultural identity, family context, and lived experience that shapes their relationship to substance use, mental health, and help-seeking. Ethical and effective care requires humility, cultural curiosity, and a readiness to adapt.

Intergenerational trauma and Indigenous healing pathways

Culture shapes how adolescents define harm, what healing looks like, and whom they trust. Indigenous youth, in particular, often carry the weight of intergenerational trauma, systemic neglect, and cultural suppression. Substance use may be deeply connected to the legacy of colonization, including boarding schools, forced relocation, and the loss of language and ceremony – disruptions that fractured families and seeded mistrust in institutions. These experiences often persist through generations in the form of disconnection, cultural loss, and emotional pain. Responding to these layers of trauma requires more than conventional talk therapy. Trauma-informed care must include culturally grounded approaches that honor Indigenous knowledge and healing traditions. Gone (2013) emphasizes that healing in Indigenous communities often involves reclaiming practices like ceremony, storytelling, and land-based healing to restore identity and belonging. These practices should never be imposed; adolescents must have real choice in whether, and how, culture becomes part of their healing. Harm reduction supports this by allowing non-coercive, identity-affirming engagement on the adolescent's terms.

Racialized stress, resistance, and community strengths

Substance use among Black and Latine youth cannot be separated from broader realities of racialized violence, economic inequality, and institutional monitoring. Many have experienced or witnessed over-policing, community trauma, school pushout, and limited access to healthcare. These systemic forces often shape a pattern of being pathologized or punished rather than supported. Culturally responsive care in this context involves naming how racism and oppression shape both risk and resilience. As Comas-Díaz et al. (2019) emphasize, racial trauma must be acknowledged directly and addressed in ways that affirm cultural identity and validate emotional responses such as protective anger as adaptive, not pathological. Healing requires approaches that frame cultural identity as a source of strength and integrate collective values, spirituality, and community connection. Protective factors such as strong family ties, faith-based support, cultural pride, and youth-led activism often emerge in these contexts. Framing these reactions as adaptive lays the groundwork for deeper trust and more sustainable therapeutic relationships.

Immigration, acculturation, and cultural role strain

For immigrant and refugee adolescents, cultural identity may be shaped by displacement, family separation, and the stress of acculturation. Many juggle adult responsibilities early on – interpreting for parents, managing finances, or caring for siblings – while trying to succeed in school and honor cultural traditions that may not align with dominant norms. Schwartz et al. (2010) describe how immigrant youth often navigate multiple social worlds, each with distinct expectations and power dynamics. This ongoing navigation creates stress but also builds under-recognized strengths and survival strategies. Culturally responsive care must acknowledge these intersecting pressures without pathologizing them. This includes identifying what is working – such as community connections or cultural identity – and supporting the adolescent's autonomy while respecting family and cultural values.

Affirmation and healing for LGBTQ+ adolescents

LGBTQ+ adolescents, especially transgender and nonbinary youth, often face profound marginalization and trauma. Experiences may include family rejection, school-based violence, community erasure, and invalidation within healthcare systems. Substance use often emerges as a coping response to chronic stress, isolation, or gender dysphoria. Harm reduction begins by creating an affirming environment where identities are accepted without question. Craig et al. (2021) found that affirming, culturally responsive care significantly improves mental health and substance use outcomes for LGBTQ+ youth, particularly when it accounts for the sociopolitical realities they face. Culturally responsive care in this context means viewing queer and trans identities as sources of resilience and creativity. It also includes recognizing the role of chosen family, online spaces, and nontraditional supports as meaningful and valid in a young person's healing process.

Spiritual identity and clinical engagement

Religious and spiritual identity can significantly shape beliefs about substance use, morality, and healing. Adolescents from Muslim, Christian, Jewish, Hindu, or Buddhist backgrounds may carry both support and stigma from their faith communities. For some, spiritual teachings provide structure and hope. For others, these same teachings may carry shame, fear, or rejection, particularly when navigating topics like drug use, sexuality, or gender identity. Post and Wade (2009) note that integrating spirituality into therapy can strengthen engagement and improve outcomes, but only when approached with openness and sensitivity. Clinicians must avoid assumptions about whether faith is helpful or harmful. Instead, they must understand how spiritual beliefs function in the adolescent's life and align treatment accordingly.

Family systems and cultural expectations

Cultural worldviews influence how adolescents and families understand behavior, responsibility, and healing. In collectivist cultures, where family harmony and interdependence are prioritized, adolescents may experience intense pressure to uphold family honor. Expressing distress or discussing substance use can be perceived as disrespectful or shameful. In many Southeast Asian communities, for example, values such as reverence for elders and emotional restraint can make it difficult for adolescents to seek support. Substance use may be viewed not as a health issue, but as a moral or relational failure. As Sue et al. (2019) emphasize, culturally responsive care requires clinicians to understand how cultural values, communication styles, and systemic oppression influence help-seeking and treatment engagement. Harm reduction in these contexts may involve redefining safer use strategies within abstinence-based households or supporting teens in navigating family expectations while maintaining personal integrity. When therapists and clients create culturally meaningful goals together, treatment becomes more relevant to the client's life and more likely to lead to lasting change.

Communication across cultural contexts

Language and communication are shaped by cultural context. Some adolescents come from communities where emotional expression is limited, direct confrontation is avoided, or mental health is not openly discussed. Others are navigating multiple languages or codes – one at home, another at school, and yet another among peers. Trickett and Jones (2007) observe that adolescents often shift communication styles depending on context, and those shifts can carry significant meaning. Culturally responsive care involves slowing down and observing how communication unfolds – noticing silences, metaphors, humor, or indirect references to pain. In multilingual households, involving interpreters or cultural brokers may be necessary, but care must be taken to protect the adolescent's privacy, dignity, and agency.

Developmental flexibility and creative engagement

Adolescents are still forming their sense of identity, and their connection to culture may be shifting. Cultural responsiveness at this stage involves avoiding assumptions, staying open, and allowing the adolescent to define what feels meaningful. Tatarsky and Kellogg (2010) highlight the value of individualized, non-coercive approaches that meet clients where they are and build goals around their readiness. Engagement strategies that include art, music, movement, or nonverbal expression can be especially effective. Session structure, language, and metaphors may need to reflect the adolescent's world. In cultures that emphasize family cohesion and respect, parallel processes with caregivers may support both individual autonomy and cultural values. Even harm reduction goals may need to shift, focusing less on substance use and more on preserving relationships, staying in school, or avoiding conflict at home.

Culturally responsive harm reduction with adolescents requires flexibility, humility, and a deep respect for the diverse ways young people make meaning of identity, connection, and change. When care is grounded in cultural context and co-created with the adolescent, healing becomes more accessible, authentic, and sustainable.

Chapter 8

Essentials of Adolescent Development and Parenting

The Adolescent Developmental Arc

We now turn our focus to how harm reduction approaches can be integrated with our scientific understanding of adolescent development and parenting styles. This synthesis helps parents create supportive, nonjudgmental, and stigma-free environments that strengthen the parent-teen relationship and equip families to navigate the challenges of adolescent substance use and mental health more effectively.

Discovering that your teen is misusing substances is disturbing, often very frightening, and fear usually compromises our best instincts on deciding how to intervene. Parenting skills are derived from a combination of our own childhood family experiences, guidance from trusted community members, and whatever self-help parenting education books we choose to read. It's easy to become confused and overwhelmed because of the many diverse "expert" opinions available.

Laurence Steinberg is a developmental psychologist whose neuroscience research and work over the past 30 years has contributed to a transformation in the way we view adolescence by underscoring the importance of viewing adolescence through a scientific lens – one that accounts for the dynamic interplay among distinct biopsychosocial and cultural factors shaping teen behavior. In his book, *The Age of Opportunity* (2014), he explains how scientific research has provided valuable insights into the neural underpinnings of substance use and addiction, offering a clearer understanding of how these behaviors develop.

Effective parenting during this stage requires a nuanced understanding of these foundational developmental processes alongside a balanced parenting style that combines warmth, responsiveness, and consistent structure. As we will see, parenting style – specifically authoritative parenting, which combines high expectations with warmth and support and aligns closely with the developmental needs of teens by providing both structure and the freedom to explore – plays a critical role in shaping adolescent outcomes. By understanding the developmental arc of adolescence and adapting their parenting style accordingly, parents can foster stronger relationships with their teens and help them build resilience, self-regulation, and decision-making skills.

Steinberg shares data showing that adolescents in the United States face more serious challenges than their peers in many other developed countries – a pattern reflected in lower academic performance, higher rates of school violence, teen pregnancy, substance use, and mental health concerns. He attributes these outcomes to systemic failures, particularly in education and parenting, where inconsistent expectations and support leave teens without the guidance they need. Adults often expect adolescents to demonstrate emotional maturity and self-regulation, while simultaneously restricting their autonomy and underestimating their competence. For Steinberg, the real crisis lies not in adolescent behavior, but in adult confusion about how to understand and support young people during this critical developmental period (Steinberg, 2014, pp. 1–3). This is reflected in our consistent finding in clinical work that parents' frustration often reflects a failure to recognize that teens are not merely smaller versions of adults but are individuals navigating a distinct developmental arc marked by significant neurological and psychological changes.

We will first discuss the range of the adolescent developmental arc and teens' vulnerability for substance use across the arc's span, and follow with exploration of parenting styles, specifically examining the importance of the authoritative parenting style. We will demonstrate how a deeper understanding of these issues can empower parents to guide teens in making healthier choices, fostering open communication, and reducing the negative consequences associated with risky behavior. Professionals working with adolescents and their families around issues of parenting will recognize that harm reduction approaches are essentially tailor-made for this developmental stage. These approaches align with what we know about adolescent growth, autonomy, and relational dynamics – topics explored in greater depth in Chapter 10.

Adolescent development is conceptually viewed as an arc, divided into stages: *early*, ages 10–14; *middle*, ages 15–17; and *late*, ages 18–24; each stage of the arc encompasses the four main spheres of human development: physical, cognitive, emotional, and social. The sidebar outlines the developmental arc, which serves as a foundation for the discussion ahead.

1. **Early Adolescence (Ages 10–14)**:
   - **Physical Development**: This stage is marked by the onset of puberty, which brings rapid physical changes such as growth spurts, development of secondary sexual characteristics (e.g., breast development in girls, voice deepening in boys), and hormonal changes.
   - **Cognitive Development**: Adolescents begin to develop more advanced reasoning skills but are still in a stage where thinking is more concrete rather than abstract. They are starting to understand cause-and-effect relationships, though they may struggle with long-term thinking and impulse control.
   - **Emotional Development**: Emotional fluctuations and mood swings are common due to hormonal changes. Self-consciousness often increases, and there's a heightened concern with body image.
   - **Social Development**: Peer relationships become increasingly important, with a shift toward seeking approval and validation from peers rather than parents. Early adolescents may also start experimenting with different social roles and exploring their identities.

2. **Middle Adolescence (Ages 15–17)**:
   - **Physical Development**: Most adolescents have gone through the major physical changes of puberty by this stage. They continue to grow physically but at a slower pace.

- **Cognitive Development**: Abstract thinking and problem-solving abilities improve. Adolescents can think hypothetically and consider multiple perspectives, but they may still struggle with risk assessment and long-term planning.
- **Emotional Development**: Identity formation becomes a central focus. Adolescents may experience conflicts with parents as they assert their independence. Romantic relationships often become more prominent.
- **Social Development**: Peer influence peaks, and adolescents may place greater importance on fitting in with specific groups. Social hierarchies and cliques often play a significant role in daily interactions. The exploration of values, goals, and personal identity deepens.

3. **Late Adolescence (Ages 18–24)**:
    - **Physical Development**: By this stage, most individuals have reached physical maturity, though the brain continues to develop into the early 20s, particularly in areas associated with decision-making and emotional regulation.
    - **Cognitive Development**: Critical thinking, planning for the future, and self-regulation continue to develop. Adolescents are better able to manage complex thoughts, engage in moral reasoning, and make long-term decisions.
    - **Emotional Development**: Emotional self-regulation improves, and young people become more emotionally stable. The focus on identity formation continues, with individuals working toward a clearer sense of self and life goals.
    - **Social Development**: Adolescents transition into adult roles, such as starting careers or higher education, forming intimate relationships, and becoming more autonomous from their families. They often experience a stronger sense of responsibility and a clearer vision of their future roles in society.

Adolescent brain plasticity: A window of opportunity and risk

Steinberg explains that understanding how the neuroplasticity of the brain – the flexible capacity of the brain's nerve cells (neurons) to change in response to experience – helps explain how and why neuroplasticity during adolescence is a critical window for brain development. This offers a unique opportunity to cultivate abilities and competencies that can contribute to long-term well-being and success in adulthood.

He also provides measurable evidence that adolescence is now about a decade long, about twice as long as in previous generations, and explains expanding the period of adolescence into the mid-twenties. The production of testosterone and estrogen at puberty accelerates plasticity and environmental sensitivity, and the wider gap between the start and end of adolescence means that young people spend more time in this state of heightened vulnerability, posing increased risks for mental health challenges and risky behavior.

Operationally, plasticity is the process through which "the outside world gets inside us and changes us [at the cellular level of the brain] allowing us to learn from experience and adapt to the environment" (Steinberg, 2014, p. 24). During this period, neural connections between various brain regions undergo significant reorganization, especially the coordination between the prefrontal cortex (the area responsible for self-regulation) and the limbic system (the brain's "sentry"), responsible for detecting rewards and threats and generating emotions. This dynamic process strengthens connections in areas that become more frequently engaged, reinforcing the neural pathways that support those specific skills, such as resisting peer pressure, controlling impulses, and thinking about long-term consequences of decisions.

A helpful analogy that Steinberg uses to explain this process in early adolescence is driving a car with an overly sensitive gas pedal and weak brakes, which makes it more difficult for teenagers to manage impulses. Eventually, later in adolescence when the brain is more organized and interconnected, the teen becomes a more "skilled driver" (Steinberg, pp. 70–71). This vulnerability offers a biological explanation for why teens who start drinking before age 14 are significantly more likely to develop substance use disorders later in life than those who wait until age 21. In fact, those who begin drinking before 14 are five times more likely to develop substance dependence at some point in their lives. Similar patterns are seen with smoking; individuals who start smoking regularly before age 18 face a much higher risk of developing nicotine addiction compared to those who start later. These findings underscore why it is so crucial for parents to limit young people's exposure to alcohol, tobacco, and other substances before age 15, when the brain is at its most vulnerable (Bava & Tapert, 2010).

Adolescence is marked by a remarkable surge in brain plasticity – far greater than in adulthood – which makes this period uniquely rich with potential and uniquely fraught with risk. The adolescent brain is wired for exploration; increases in novelty-seeking and curiosity are not just quirks of development, but adaptive features designed to maximize learning while the brain is most malleable. But this openness to experience is a double-edged sword. The same plasticity that supports rapid cognitive and emotional growth also leaves the brain especially vulnerable to harm. Mental health challenges, which are relatively rare before age 10, begin to rise sharply in adolescence, and while those who reach their mid-20s without developing a disorder are statistically more resilient, the adolescent years remain a critical window of vulnerability. Negative influences – whether psychological stressors, substance use, or physical trauma like concussions – can have outsized impacts during this time, with adolescent brains shown to be more susceptible to injury than those of adults (CDC, 2022). In short, adolescence is both a time of extraordinary opportunity and considerable risk – a developmental good news/bad news story.

Building on this, while adult brains retain some capacity for change, the adolescent brain's plasticity is far more dynamic and expansive. With these wide-open windows for learning and adaptation, what enters during this period – experiences, relationships, habits – matters immensely. The surge in novelty-seeking and curiosity so characteristic of adolescence isn't random; it's an evolutionary strategy designed to capitalize on this heightened plasticity, encouraging young people to explore, experiment, and absorb as much as possible while the brain is primed for growth.

The Developmental Arc and Substance Use

The developmental arc comprises six main themes of adolescent maturation:

- Physical and brain development
- Identity formation and autonomy
- Peer influence and social development

- Emotional and stress-related factors
- Family and environmental factors
- Cognitive development and moral reasoning.

The themes reflect a combination of dynamically interactive variables that can create a perfect storm increasing susceptibility to drug use. Harm reduction approaches align with the developmental arc by providing a supportive scaffolding that respects teens' autonomy, recognizes the influence of their social environment, and addresses the realities of their cognitive and emotional development. By focusing on minimizing harm and encouraging open communication, these strategies offer adolescents a path to healthier choices that coincide with their developmental needs, supporting their journey toward becoming informed, responsible adults.

What follows is an overview of each theme and suggestions for implementing harm reduction-inspired early interventions for reducing the impact of substance use.

Brain development and risk-taking

As we reviewed earlier in this chapter, the open window of neuroplasticity during adolescence, especially in the prefrontal cortex and the limbic system, is a work in progress until the mid-20s. In early adolescence, this window makes kids more prone to impulsive behavior and risk-taking. Also, the brain's reward system, especially the release of dopamine, is particularly active during adolescence which explains why teens are drawn to experiences that provide immediate pleasure or reward. Moving through adolescence, coordination between the prefrontal cortex and limbic system improves as the neural circuits (aka "wiring") become more organized so by the time we leave puberty and the window closes, plasticity is traded for organizational efficiency.

Addressing risk-taking and impulsivity

Harm reduction-based education on safer substance use and the potential consequences, can help adolescents make informed choices while acknowledging that some will engage in risk-taking behavior regardless of abstinence messages. In middle and late adolescence, harm reduction-inspired approaches like providing safe spaces for discussions about drug use, can mitigate the impact of impulsive decisions. Programs that promote safe practices, such as using sterile equipment or setting limits, resonate with adolescents who may still struggle with impulse control and long-term planning.

Identity formation and autonomy

Throughout adolescence, individuals wrestle with questions about who they are, what they believe, and where they fit in the world. Erik Erikson (1968) described this as the "Identity versus Role Confusion" stage, where successful resolution leads to a strong sense of personal identity. As adolescents strive for independence from their parents, they may experiment with drugs as a way of asserting control over their own choices. This can be part of their broader quest to form an identity and establish autonomy. Adolescents often try different behaviors and roles as they explore their identities. Substance use can sometimes be seen as a way to fit into a certain group, experiment with new experiences, or rebel against authority.

Supporting identity formation and autonomy

Harm reduction aligns with adolescents' developmental need for autonomy by giving them *choices* rather than imposing strict abstinence. This approach empowers teens to make decisions based on their values and goals, which is crucial as they explore their identity. Adolescents in middle and late adolescence are particularly sensitive to judgment and authority. Harm reduction approaches that offer respectful, nonjudgmental support allow teens to feel understood and validated as they navigate their choices, helping them to make healthier decisions without feeling alienated.

Peer influence and social development

Since social acceptance and peer relationships become extremely important during adolescence, teens may feel pressure to use drugs to fit in with their peer group or to be seen as "cool" or adventurous. Their concern with impression management often influences them to try drugs to enhance their social image or to conform to perceived expectations, especially if drug use is normalized or glamorized in their social circles.

Steinberg describes this as the *peer effect*, the tendency for teens to be more likely to engage in risky behavior when they are with peers compared to when they are alone. The peer effect is linked to the brain's heightened activity in the reward system, increasing kids' sensitivity to social rewards and approval from peers. This increased activation encourages behaviors that might gain peer approval, even if risky (Steinberg, 2014, pp. 92–93).

Engaging with peer influence and social dynamics

To meet teens where they are at, harm reduction involves peer education, where teens learn from other young people about safer substance use practices. This can increase the credibility and relevance of harm reduction messages among adolescents. Harm reduction strategies often involve creating spaces where teens can socialize without the pressure to use substances. Programs that facilitate drug-free events or support healthier ways of coping with peer pressure can be effective, particularly as adolescents prioritize peer relationships.

Emotional and stress-related factors

Adolescents' capacity for self-regulation – the ability to control impulses, delay gratification, and manage emotions – is a key predictor of long-term well-being. As works in progress, to a teen, using substances might seem like an appealing way to escape from negative emotions or to enhance positive ones. Because adolescents are more likely to use substances as a coping mechanism for dealing with stress, anxiety, or depression, substances might be used to self-medicate or to experiment with altering their mood states to help them try to balance their heightened emotional sensitivity and fluctuations due to hormonal changes.

Enhancing emotional regulation and coping skills

Teaching alternative coping strategies, such as mindfulness or stress management, can help them regulate their emotions more effectively. Harm reduction approaches empower teens, facilitating the learning of skills to increase self-awareness, manage stress and resist peer pressure, and equipping them with tools to handle these challenging situations in healthier ways.

Family and environmental factors

Our families are responsible for transmitting the culture of the communities we live in to our children. Each family has its own particular lens and filter and so we learn from them how anger is expressed and conflicts are managed, and how emotions like love and affection are expressed. If the environment of the family normalizes drug use and it is present, teens may be more likely to experiment with substances themselves (Nawi et al., 2021). Adolescents with easy access to substances in their schools may have a higher risk of trying them. As we discuss in Chapter 5, zero-tolerance expectations by parents will usually increase the likelihood of use and less safe use. Researchers like Steinberg have been able to rule out one common stigmatizing misconception – that early substance use is simply a byproduct of personality traits like impulsivity or poor self-control. While it is true that impulsivity can play a role, both animal and human studies suggest that drug exposure during adolescence itself has a unique impact on brain development and behavior, beyond personality traits or individual choice (Cadet et al., 2018).

Promoting family and community involvement

Educating parents on how to communicate openly and effectively with their teens about substance use can strengthen family bonds and help adolescents feel supported in their choices. We discuss specific skills training for parents when we review CRAFT (Community Reinforcement and Family Training) in Chapter 12. Parents can support this development by offering guidance, setting boundaries, and helping their children develop emotional regulation skills. Also, by involving community resources, harm reduction creates a supportive environment that fosters positive development, offering adolescents access to mentors, healthcare providers, and social workers who can guide them through their developmental stages.

Cognitive development and moral reasoning

As adolescents move through late adolescence and their ability to think abstractly increases, they start to question societal norms and experiment with behaviors considered taboo, including drug use. Because of the usual lag in impulse regulation, they may still struggle to fully assess the long-term consequences of drug use, focusing instead on the potential rewards, making it harder to make informed choices regarding substances.

Providing science-based resources to mitigate cognitive deficits

Harm reduction education provides honest information about both risks and safer use practices, which is critical for teens whose cognitive development still makes them susceptible to risky behaviors. Harm reduction education programs are transparent about the immediate and long-term effects of drug use and often offer access to resources like counseling and healthcare services. This is especially important for adolescents who may be more open to seeking help if they feel their choices are respected rather than judged.

Parenting Styles and Harm Reduction

A well-established body of literature on effective parenting and parenting education has been developed over the past 60 years and can be traced to the foundational research by developmental psychologist Diane Baumrind (1966). She identified three main parenting styles –Authoritarian, Authoritative, and Permissive – and the Neglectful style has since been added by other researchers (Maccoby, & Martin, 1983). These styles, which describe how parents interact with their children and how they manage discipline and communication, have been incorporated into the work of child, couple, and family therapists as well as parent educators since then.

For context, the sidebar provides an overview of parenting styles – from Baumrind's original typology to later refinements – which underpins the discussion of how these styles intersect with harm reduction principles.

1. **Authoritarian Parenting**:
   - **Characteristics**: Authoritarian parents are highly demanding but not very responsive. They have strict rules and expectations, enforce discipline through punishment, and offer little warmth or feedback to their children.
   - **Outcomes**: Children raised with this style may be obedient and proficient, but they might also develop lower self-esteem and social competence, and higher levels of anxiety.

2. **Authoritative Parenting**:
   - **Characteristics**: This style is marked by a balance between responsiveness and demandingness. Authoritative parents set clear rules and guidelines but are also responsive to their children's needs and are willing to explain the reasons behind rules.
   - **Outcomes**: Children of authoritative parents tend to be independent, self-regulated, and socially competent. This style is often associated with positive outcomes in child and adolescent development.

3. **Permissive Parenting**:
   - **Characteristics**: Permissive parents are highly responsive but not demanding. They set few boundaries or rules and are lenient, often acting more like a friend than a parent.
   - **Outcomes**: Children of permissive parents may struggle with self-discipline, may be more self-centered, and may have difficulty in authority-based environments such as school.

4. **Neglectful (Uninvolved) Parenting**:
   - **Characteristics**: This style is characterized by low responsiveness and low demandingness. Neglectful parents are uninvolved in their child's life, providing little guidance, attention, or support.
   - **Outcomes**: Children with neglectful parents often suffer from a lack of self-control, have low self-esteem, and may struggle academically and socially.

Authoritarian Parenting: Authoritarian parents are very demanding but not very responsive to their children's needs. They have strict rules and expectations and use punishment to enforce discipline and offer little warmth or validating feedback to their children. This style raises children who are often obedient and accomplished, but they are prone to lower self-esteem, uncertain social skills, and higher levels of anxiety. Children will be compliant when they feel threatened but often respond with aggression and oppositional behavior.

Authoritative Parenting: This style is characterized by a balance between responsiveness and demandingness. These parents establish clear rules and guidelines but are also responsive to their children's needs and are willing to explain the reasons behind rules. Children of authoritative parents are more likely to have higher levels of self-efficacy, are more responsible and socially competent. They tend to be more skilled with their emotional regulation.

Permissive Parenting: Permissive parents are highly responsive but not demanding. They set few boundaries or rules and are lenient, often acting more like a friend than a parent. Children of permissive parents may struggle with self-discipline and behavioral impulsivity, be more self-centered, and may have difficulty in authority-based environments such as school. "Enabling" is a pejorative label commonly given to more permissive parents by one-size-fits-all treatment programs and 12-step mutual help programs.

Neglectful (Uninvolved) Parenting: This style is characterized by low responsiveness and low demandingness. Neglectful parents are uninvolved in their child's life, providing little guidance, attention, or support. Children with neglectful parents often suffer from a lack of self-control, have low self-esteem, and may struggle academically and socially (difficulty forming nurturing relationships, self-reliance out of necessity, less effective coping strategies).

Harm Reduction Embraces Authoritative Parenting

Parenting styles fall along a range that captures differences in control, flexibility, boundaries, and expectations – spanning from the most rigid (authoritarian) to the most disengaged (neglectful/uninvolved), with authoritative parenting representing a balanced middle ground.

Laurence Steinberg's *The Ten Basic Principles of Good Parenting* (2005) was a significant contribution to confirming that authoritative parenting is a balanced style. That it creates a nurturing and structured environment that fosters healthy development across emotional, social, and cognitive domains, making it widely regarded as most effective for fostering self-regulation, academic success, and emotional well-being in adolescents.

Effective parenting during adolescence requires balancing structure with responsiveness, mirroring the principles of authoritative parenting. This approach acknowledges the developmental arc of adolescence as a time of heightened risk-taking, emotional volatility, and identity formation. Risk-taking and challenging authority, for example, are not merely disruptive behaviors but are essential components of the process through which teens establish autonomy and self-identity. Recognizing these behaviors as part of a normal developmental trajectory allows parents to respond with guidance and empathy, rather than judgment or rigidity.

The balance in authoritative parenting is more likely to be attained by establishing clear rules and expectations with warmth, support, and open communication. This balance helps children understand boundaries while feeling loved and valued. Ideally, this encourages independent thinking while still respecting rules and guidelines.

Long before harm reduction was formally recognized as a viable psychosocial intervention, psychologists Stanton Peele and Robert J. Meyers were independently incorporating harm reduction principles into their work – particularly through approaches grounded in authoritative parenting. Peele is a prominent advocate of the personal responsibility and choice model of addiction, emphasizing the role of individual agency and self-regulation in recovery. He has long promoted preventive parenting strategies as a means of reducing substance-related harm. Meyers, meanwhile, developed CRAFT (Community Reinforcement and Family Training), an evidence-based intervention that supports families and loved ones of people who use substances (Smith & Meyers, 2023). Both models draw from authoritative parenting frameworks, reflecting the developmental research of Diana Baumrind (1966) and Laurence Steinberg (2014), and aim to equip parents with the skills to set clear boundaries, maintain strong relationships, and support self-directed change.

Authoritative Parenting and the Developmental Tasks of Adolescence

Peele, in his book *How to Addiction Proof Your Child* (2007), identified goals for parents to best promote their children's well-being by essentially incorporating an authoritative parenting style to allow parents to become de facto *addiction prevention agents*. He suggests ways that parents can act as prevention agents in reviewing some of the important adolescent maturation results.

Developing self-control and responsibility

Studies show that children raised by authoritative parents – those who combine warmth and responsiveness with clear boundaries – are less likely to engage in delinquent behavior, substance misuse, or other risky activities (Steinberg, 2014; Peele, 2007). Authoritative parenting is consistent but flexible, reducing confusion and helping children understand the expectations and consequences of their behavior. Authoritative parents explain the reasons behind rules and discipline and their children are encouraged to think critically about their actions and its impact on others.

Fostering a sense of independence and accountability enables teens to better resist peer pressure and unhealthy habits. While teens should have freedom to grow, parents need to set firm boundaries regarding substance use and risky behaviors. Consistency in enforcing these rules helps teens understand the importance of safety and respect. Peele emphasizes that addiction *prevention* starts with teaching children self-regulation and responsibility from a young age.

Creating strong emotional bonds

Parenting authoritatively means that parents are attuned to their children's unique emotional needs, and adapt their parenting style accordingly. This child-centered approach fosters a strong sense of security and self-esteem in children, helping them feel understood and supported. Children raised this way tend to develop better emotional regulation skills because they are encouraged to express their feelings and learn how to manage them appropriately. Peele encouraged parents to help their children learn how to cope with stress, make good decisions, and set limits for themselves.

Building confidence and competence

Authoritative parents provide a supportive environment that encourages learning and curiosity, helping their children build competence in various areas of life, such as academics, hobbies, or sports. This often translates to better academic performance because children feel motivated and supported in their educational endeavors.

Peele embraces the authoritative parenting value of setting high standards and helping children understand the value of discipline and hard work. This fosters intrinsic motivation, leading to better academic outcomes. And children who feel confident in their abilities are less likely to turn to substances as a way to escape feelings of inadequacy.

Fostering healthy relationships

Competent social skills are more likely to be developed in authoritative parenting homes where communication is more open. Healthier relationships are formed when children learn how to interact with others respectfully and assertively. Peele advises parents to be transparent about emotions, life challenges, and specifically drugs, reducing the stigma normally surrounding the topic. A supportive, communicative family culture allows children to feel more secure and reduces their need to seek out substances or risky behaviors as coping mechanisms.

Peele goes a step further and argues that social connections and healthy friendships are key in inoculating children, so to speak, against addiction. Those with strong relationships and positive parental role models are more likely to develop empathy and cooperative behaviors and less likely to seek out unhealthy behaviors.

Developing a sense of purpose and personal fulfillment

Authoritative parents play an important role in helping their child develop a sense of purpose, which can serve as a protective factor against risky behaviors, including substance use. A strong sense of purpose gives children a reason to engage meaningfully with the world, helping them build resilience, self-worth, and motivation to pursue fulfilling goals.

Empowering parents to discuss substance use without fear

The increased trust and emotional safety in families with an authoritative parenting culture enables parents to more effectively be prevention agents by having often-difficult conversations about substance use without fear. Rather than using scare tactics, Peele advises parents to educate their children about drugs and alcohol in a factual and calm manner. The goal is to create a realistic understanding of the risks and consequences without driving curiosity or rebellion. Parents are encouraged to educate themselves with science-based information about substance use so they can be more comfortable in discussing addiction openly and provide their children with the tools to recognize the signs of problematic behavior in themselves and others.

One of Peele's core beliefs is that addiction arises when people turn to substances as a way to cope with life's challenges. Therefore, parents teaching children healthy coping skills for stress reduction, frustration, and disappointment, is vital for his goal of "addiction-proofing" their children.

Social Media's Impact on Adolescent Development

The widespread adoption of smartphones in the early 2010s has profoundly shaped how adolescents engage with developmental tasks and milestones. A central challenge for parents today is managing their children's use of social media platforms that increasingly influence identity formation, peer dynamics, and emotional health.

Social psychologist Jonathan Haidt (2024) describes excessive smartphone and social media use among youth as a public health crisis. While acknowledging some benefits of social media, **Twenge et al. (2022)** have linked rising rates of anxiety, depression, self-harm, and suicide – particularly among girls – to social media's amplification of exclusion, rumor-spreading, and appearance-based comparisons on platforms like Instagram and TikTok. Haidt also emphasizes how these platforms are intentionally designed to be addictive, employing operant conditioning strategies such as variable rewards – intermittent likes, notifications, and algorithmic feedback – that mirror gambling mechanics. These features drive compulsive engagement, fostering behavioral patterns that resemble addictions to food, shopping, or internet use (Haidt, (2024).

As discussed in Chapter 6, harm reduction frames addiction as a pattern of compulsive behavior that overrides impulse control and judgment. This makes adolescents – whose neurodevelopmental immaturity limits self-regulation – especially vulnerable to social media overuse. Excessive screen time displaces key developmental activities like face-to-face interaction, exercise, and sleep. It can delay social skill development and emotional regulation, increase isolation, and elevate risks for anxiety, depression, and low self-esteem. Moreover, teens are more exposed to peer modeling of risky behaviors – including substance use – which may reinforce self-medicating patterns and habitual digital escape.

Unsupervised free play and the role of authoritative parenting

Haidt and Lukianoff (2021), Peele (2007), and Steinberg (2014) all highlight the developmental costs of modern childhood's loss of unsupervised free play – self-directed, unstructured activities where children explore and problem-solve without adult control. Free play cultivates independence, creativity, social competence, and an internal locus of control. Without it, children lose vital opportunities to build resilience, navigate challenges, and develop confidence through natural consequences.

Contemporary barriers – digital surveillance, safety fears, urban environments, and legal scrutiny – make unsupervised play harder to access. The presence of smartphones introduces new risks, from cyberbullying to location tracking, even in outdoor settings. Overly structured schedules and social norms about constant supervision further limit children's autonomy. Haidt and Peele echo Steinberg's concern that excessive adult control undermines resilience. In contrast, authoritative parenting – characterized by warmth, guidance, and high expectations – strikes a developmentally optimal balance. By encouraging autonomy within clear limits, this parenting style supports healthy risk-taking and learning. When parents model emotional regulation and provide room for mistakes, they help their children grow into adaptable, confident adolescents.

Encouragingly, Haidt's research and advocacy have helped spur policy efforts worldwide. For example, Australia has passed legislation banning social media for those under 16 and requiring platform-based age verification (Australian Government, 2024). As of early 2025, several U.S. states have introduced legislation aimed at regulating minors' access to social media, reflecting growing concern about online safety and mental health. Laws such as Utah's Social Media Regulation Act and California's Age-Appropriate Design Code require parental consent, age verification, and child-focused privacy protections, though many face legal challenges over enforcement (California Age-Appropriate Design Code Act, 2022; Utah S.B. 152,

2023). Other proposals aim to delay smartphone access until age 14, restrict school-time phone use, and promote offline activities like free play (Wait Until 8th, n.d.).

Recognizing that individual families can't enforce limits alone, Haidt (2023) encourages collective parental action – collaborative norms that reduce peer pressure and create consistency across households. Delaying access, promoting offline play, and setting shared expectations can mitigate social media's risks and support stronger emotional development. While digital challenges are real, they can be managed through education, boundaries, and community support. Through informed, collective strategies, families and communities can help adolescents develop the emotional and social resilience needed to thrive in a digital world.

Chapter 9

Why HRT Works Well with Adolescents

In our discussion of the National Harm Reduction Coalition's (NHRC) eight basic tenets of harm reduction in Chapter 1 (also Appendix A), we describe how the principles embrace the philosophy that harm reduction is based on our knowledge that human beings naturally will engage in behaviors that carry risks. Harm reduction values each person's uniqueness, individuality, and dignity, and respects their right to make choices. This shifts the focus from attempting to restrict or prohibit risky behaviors to reducing the negative consequences associated with them. Risk-taking, challenging authority, and novelty-seeking are normal teen behaviors that are often part of a process of establishing autonomy and identity. This is often reflected by their irrational behavior, poor judgment, emotional dysregulation, and problems with impulse control.

Harm reduction is nonjudgmental and is person- and family-centered at its core. It views people as *whole* people, never defining them in the context of their substance use. Adolescents are siblings, students, peers, musicians, athletes, and employees with unique skills and personalities who may also use substances. This wider lens perspective of viewing substance use as being a *part* of a teen's life enables them to more readily identify the various paths to well-being for each person. It appreciates that experimentation with drugs – sometimes including unwise, excessive, or dangerous use – occurs in a context where the vast majority of drug use does not lead to addiction problems.

Being client-centered encourages counselors to collaborate with individuals and families in making goals for behavioral changes, thereby empowering teens and meeting them where they are at. Self-empowerment helps counter the shame and stigma of substance use and thereby lowers a common barrier to engaging in treatment. Harm reduction approaches are more likely to successfully engage young people in treatment because people in emotional pain, when shown compassion and given a stigma-free environment, are more willing to open up and share their worries and concerns.

Harm Reduction Tenets Parallel Adolescent Development

The tenets that comprise the foundation pieces of harm reduction treatment strategies are compatible with adolescent development, as they complement the normal adolescent developmental dynamics of risk-taking, autonomy-building, and decision-making that characterize this stage of life.

As reviewed in Chapter 8, teens are at a developmental disadvantage when evaluating the risks and rewards involved in making choices, because their impulse control and ability to weigh short- and long-term risks and rewards are a work in progress. When substance use is involved in the equation, young peoples' difficulty in seeing future costs often offers the immediacy of getting high as seemingly the best choice. This challenge is compounded by the nature of addictive substances, which tend to provide immediate benefits but delayed costs.

HRT shifts adolescent maladaptive learning into adaptive growth

A common denominator in working with all teens is to facilitate their learning to make choices that will more readily shift from maladaptive choices to choices that are adaptive to psychological well-being. Teens are at a developmental disadvantage when evaluating the risks and rewards involved in decision-making because their impulse control and ability to weigh short- and long-term consequences are still developing.

Rather than solely focusing on abstinence, harm reduction approaches aim to minimize the negative consequences of drug use. Their flexibility and dynamism allow for a more collaborative relationship with young people, inviting them to explore what needs they are fulfilling by using substances, the risks involved, and what is required to make meaningful changes.

The dynamic adaptive learning approach more accurately reflects a young person's unfolding developmental trajectory and offers greater flexibility and treatment options than the static disease approach. In this treatment environment, framing drug use as a choice within their control encourages teens to engage in discussions about options for coping with urges. HRT focuses on helping them understand their cravings, anticipate and manage the impulse to use, and work through the underlying issues that substance use temporarily alleviates (Lessin, 2023a; Szalavitz, 2016).

This perspective fosters greater engagement in treatment, particularly for those with more problematic use, and helps keep them in treatment longer. Teens are more willing to collaborate in their care when their shortcomings and failures aren't reinforced, and when they feel genuinely invested in the process of change. Viewed in this way, young people gain a clearer understanding of the harms associated with their substance use and become more willing to take steps toward change.

Acknowledges the importance of the structural contexts of families

Harm reduction recognizes the importance of the unique structural and contextual variables of the environment and communities each person lives in. Families provide the infrastructure for transmitting culture and values to its members, and so working with families whenever possible will increase the likelihood of effecting change with adolescents. Family therapist pioneer Virginia Satir (1964) used the analogy of a baby's mobile to demonstrate the dynamic nature of families and the importance of recognizing how interconnected and interdependent family members are.

For example, if there is a stress to one part of the mobile – a job change, an illness, or emotional crisis – all other parts need to adjust to maintain balance. Just as a mobile is sensitive to small changes in movement, families will adjust to small shifts in behavior, roles, or communication patterns. Mobiles have parts of varying size and weights and despite the differences of each person in a family, they all co-exist together as a unit. Flexibility is important in mobiles and families, helping to adapt to changes and challenges while maintaining their integrity.

Consider a family where one parent believes in strict consequences for misbehavior, such as taking away privileges immediately, while the other parent prefers a more lenient, discussion-based approach. Their teenage son, Jimmy, quickly picks up on this inconsistency. When he stays out past curfew, his mother grounds him for a week, but his father secretly lets him go out after a couple of days, believing the punishment was too harsh. Sensing this divide, Jimmy begins playing his parents against each other, telling his dad that his mom is being unfair and exaggerating how strict she is, while telling his mom that his dad "already said it was fine" when she tries to enforce rules. Over time, their inconsistent discipline creates chaos and resentment, leading to frequent arguments between the parents, a loss of parental authority, and Jimmy learning that rules are negotiable based on which parent he asks.

To restore balance – like adjusting a mobile – the parents decide to compromise on a unified approach. They initially try a middle-ground discipline plan, agreeing to a shorter consequence with a discussion about expectations. However, when Jimmy continues testing boundaries, they realize their first approach isn't working as well as they had hoped. Instead of giving up or reverting to old patterns, they decide to experiment with a different strategy – adding logical consequences, such as Jimmy needing to check in more frequently when he's out, rather than just grounding him.

Over time, they tweak their approach through trial and error, learning what works best for their family dynamic. As they become more consistent and flexible in their responses, Jimmy stops seeing opportunities for manipulation and begins respecting the rules more. Their adjustments don't happen overnight, but by staying open to change and working together, they create a more balanced and effective approach to discipline. Like a mobile adjusting to external forces, the family regains stability through patience, adaptability, and a shared commitment to problem-solving together.

Addiction as a complex biopsychosocial phenomenon

Addiction, from a harm reduction perspective, is understood as a complex interplay of biological, psychological, and social/environmental factors unique to each individual (Zinberg, 1986). Building on this understanding, harm reduction views substance use as existing on a continuum – from no use to hazardous/chaotic use – and emphasizes personalized strategies to reduce harm at any point along that spectrum (Figure 1.1, page 7) This is in contrast to the preponderance of one-size-fits-all abstinent-only treatment programs and mutual help groups (Alcoholics Anonymous [AA], Narcotics Anonymous [NA]) that rely mostly on disease models of addiction (Paquette et al., 2022).

The etiology of addiction remains a subject of ongoing debate, with models ranging from NIDA's chronic, relapsing brain disease framework (Volkow & Koob, 2015), and the medical/spiritual models of AA and NA (Alcoholics Anonymous, 2001), to SAMHSA's biopsychosocial approach (Substance Abuse and Mental Health Services Administration, 2020). Other influential perspectives include the self-medication models of Edward Khantzian (1997) and Gabor Maté (2010), the personal responsibility and choice models advanced by Stanton Peele (Peele & Brodsky, 1975) and Gene Heyman (2009), and the social context model of Bruce Alexander (2008).

The disease model of treatment makes adolescents particularly vulnerable in a number of ways. Teenagers often come to treatment very reluctantly, so telling them they have "a disease", as is common in traditional treatment programs, can undermine their existing emotional vulnerabilities, hampering whatever motivation they may have to get well. Instead, harm reduction approaches are informed by counseling psychology (American Psychological Association, n.d.) and based on human developmental (Erikson, 1950) and attachment theories (Ainsworth et al., 1978; Bowlby, 1988). Rather than pathologizing behavior, these models emphasize lifespan growth and early relational bonds as the foundation for emotional and social development across life. In other words, people have "problems in living" and that the challenges we face are normal ones as we move through our lives in predictable developmental stages. In addition, a study led by William Miller, the developer of MI, found two client factors as optimally predictive of resumed drinking: lack of coping skills and belief in the disease model of alcoholism (Miller & Rollnick, 2012).

Another problem with applying the disease model to adolescents is that it relies on substance use disorder (SUD) diagnoses as the foundation for treatment planning. This approach raises concerns about pathologizing what may be normative adolescent behaviors, which can inadvertently reinforce stigma and exacerbate already low self-esteem (Levine, 2013). While diagnostic labels can serve a practical function – guiding treatment recommendations or providing a shared shorthand among providers – they tend to emphasize substance use as the central problem, often at the expense of understanding and treating underlying mental health issues such as anxiety, depression, trauma, or ADHD, as the author has previously discussed (Lessin, 2023a). Perhaps most importantly, these labels often fail to capture the individuality of the teen and the complexity of their family, cultural, and developmental context (Lessin, 2023b).

These limitations are further amplified by structural and systemic pressures. Insurance reimbursement policies often require clinicians to assign a formal psychiatric diagnosis in order to justify care, forcing providers to reduce nuanced and overlapping experiences into discrete, billable categories. This pressure can result in treatment that is diagnostically driven rather than developmentally or contextually informed. The challenge is compounded by the fact that mental health and addiction services are frequently siloed – that is, separated into distinct funding and service delivery systems with minimal coordination – despite the high rates of co-occurring mental health and substance use disorders (California Health Care Foundation, 2022). As CHCF notes, this fragmentation leads to delayed care, poor communication between providers, and gaps in treatment, often leaving one aspect of a teen's experience unaddressed. These systemic failures contribute to poorer outcomes, including increased hospitalizations, school disruptions, justice involvement, and long-term disengagement from care. Counselors, caught between clinical ethics and reimbursement demands, may find themselves prioritizing the diagnosis that fits most neatly within the DSM framework rather than treating the full person. Ultimately, this limits both the accuracy of diagnosis and the accessibility of integrated, developmentally appropriate care (Barry et al., 2014).

Instead, harm reduction informs us that we need a treatment model that reflects a young person's unfolding developmental trajectory, offering holistic and flexible options based on the teen's wishes. Treatment from this perspective focuses on collaboratively helping teens understand their urges to get high, anticipate and better manage impulses to use substances, and work through any underlying issues that are being temporarily solved by getting high. People of all ages are far more open to collaborating in a treatment process that doesn't reinforce shortcomings and failures, and when they feel invested in the process of change. In this treatment environment, we nonjudgmentally frame drug use as a choice – one that a person can have control over – and foster discussions of different options for coping, both with urges to use and with life challenges.

HRT empowers youth by connecting with where they are in their process of change. They are more likely to engage in treatment in an atmosphere of mutual respect and safety, offering them an opportunity to share openly and honestly about themselves and explore the possibility of making positive changes and living well without relying on drugs. Pioneering harm reduction advocate Dan Bigg introduced the idea of "any positive change" as a form of progress and success with people who use substances if it helps to increase the motivation to change, especially with adolescents (Bigg, 2001).

Mediating harms with reality-based drug education

The potential for tragic harm when using certain drugs requires that reality-based drug information be offered to people who use substances, especially adolescents, given how normal adolescent development includes the tendency to distrust and challenge authority. Teens will respond more positively when the information is scientifically accurate, presented honestly, interactively, and nonjudgmentally with the focus on *safety* instead of only abstinence. They want to feel mutual respect so that they will make up their own minds about safety (Drug Policy Alliance, 2023). Unfortunately, most schools in the United States are abstinence-based, and therefore foster cynicism among teenagers about any drug information shared by adults (Kumar et al., 2013) We discussed drug education programs earlier in this book – see Chapter 4 for a deeper look.

The Spectrum of Substance Use in Adolescence

Many teens have used alcohol and other drugs without misusing or experiencing significant harms. Their use can be categorized into different patterns based on frequency, intention, and consequences. Harm reduction describes use on a spectrum – from none to experimental, to sporadic/occasional, to regular, to problematic, to hazardous or chaotic use (see Figure 1.1) To deepen understanding of the spectrum of substance use, Exercise 3 offers a guided opportunity to explore how patterns of use can vary in terms of frequency, intention, and impact.

No Use: The teen has not used any alcohol or other drugs. This may reflect personal, cultural, or familial values, lack of opportunity, or simply a developmental stage where experimentation has not occurred. It is important to note that "no use" does not necessarily imply greater resilience or lower risk – it is one point along a fluid spectrum of behavior that may change over time.

Experimental Use: Curious about effects of drugs or use when invited to with people the teen is with; Use just a few times without keeping a supply. Examples are:

- A 16-year-old tries cannabis at a party out of curiosity but does not use it again.
- A 15-year-old takes a sip of alcohol at a family gathering because older siblings offer it.
- A high school student tries a friend's ADHD medication once to see if it helps them focus on studying.

Consequences associated with experimental use usually have minimal impact on school, relationships, or health.

- A teen tries alcohol once and experiences mild nausea but no significant consequences.
- A student smokes cannabis once and feels anxious, deciding not to try it again.
- A 15-year-old takes a friend's ADHD medication and has trouble sleeping and does not repeat the behavior.

Sporadic/Occasional Use: Substance use is situational and tied to specific events, social settings, or desired effects. The individual does not use habitually or feel compelled to use when substances are available but may engage for enjoyment, relaxation, or enhancement of an experience. This pattern carries lower immediate risk but could lead to increased use depending on context and personal factors. Examples are:

- A 17-year-old drinks alcohol only at special events, like birthdays or prom.
- A teenager smokes cannabis with friends once every few months but doesn't seek it out.
- A high school athlete vapes nicotine on weekends but does not use it daily.

Examples of consequences associated with sporadic/occasional use involve increased risk, are situational, and include occasional poor decision-making (e.g., impaired judgment, skipping class), parental discipline or minor school consequences. They also involve an increased chance of exposure to riskier substances or peer pressure.

- A 17-year-old drinks alcohol at parties and once gets caught by parents, leading to temporary grounding.
- A teen smokes cannabis monthly, once getting too high and missing a school assignment.
- A high school athlete vapes nicotine on weekends and develops a mild cough but doesn't see it as a problem.

Regular Use: Substance use follows a developing routine and serves as a coping mechanism for stress, social anxiety, or relaxation. Use occurs both alone and socially, with the individual actively obtaining substances. While no significant impact on functioning may be observed, the behavior is beginning to raise concern, with occasional or minimal risk-taking present. Examples are:

- A 16-year-old smokes cannabis a few times a week to help with stress.
- A student takes an Adderall pill before most exams, believing it helps them perform better.
- A teen drinks alcohol every weekend with friends and feels it's part of their social routine.
- A college freshman microdoses psilocybin mushrooms multiple times a week, believing it helps with creativity and focus but struggles to concentrate on schoolwork when not using.

Consequences of regular substance use during adolescence can impact mental health, physical well-being, academic performance, and relationships. These effects often develop gradually and are not always immediately linked to the substance use itself, making them easy to overlook. Over time, ongoing use can contribute to decreased motivation, difficulty concentrating, disrupted sleep, increased anxiety or mood swings, strained family or peer relationships, and higher risk-taking behavior. Some common examples include:

- Regular cannabis use affects motivation and focus, contributing to a noticeable drop in grades.
- Repeated Adderall use before exams can lead to psychological dependence, sleep disruption, and heightened anxiety.
- Increased alcohol consumption may result in impaired judgment and driving under the influence, sometimes leading to accidents or legal trouble.

- Using psychedelics like mushrooms in unsafe or unpredictable settings raises the risk of intense psychological distress or engaging in unsafe behavior.

Examples of consequences associated with regular use are: cannabis use frequency affects motivation, contributing to a drop in grades; Adderall taken before most exams becoming reliant on it for studying, leading to increased anxiety and insomnia; increased drinking leads to driving under the influence resulting in minor car accident; using mushrooms in unsafe environments, increasing the likelihood of experiencing distress or engaging in risky behaviors

Problematic Use: Frequent, often solitary substance use that is outside the norm of one's peer group. The individual is actively seeking out substances, leading to noticeable declines in physical, psychological, social, and academic functioning. Increased risk-taking behaviors are present, and substance use is beginning to interfere with daily life. Examples are:

- A 16-year-old starts vaping nicotine multiple times a day and feels irritable when they can't.
- A teen who used to drink only on weekends now drinks several times a week.
- A high school student begins using cannabis every morning before school to "take the edge off" and struggles to stop.
- A college sophomore home from school steals prescription pills from a family member to use recreationally.
- A previously high-achieving student starts missing assignments and cutting classes because they're too tired or hungover.

These patterns of use are often associated with the following escalating consequences:

- **Emotional dysregulation**: The teen who vapes daily becomes increasingly irritable and anxious when access is limited, making emotional regulation and focus more difficult.
- **Academic decline and increased risk-taking**: The student who now drinks on school nights begins falling behind in coursework and is caught coming to school intoxicated.
- **Compulsive use and dependence**: The teen who uses cannabis each morning starts to rely on it just to function, and skipping a day leads to withdrawal symptoms and decreased school performance.
- **Legal and family consequences**: The college student who steals prescription pills risks criminal charges and loses trust within their family.
- **Loss of academic and extracurricular opportunities**: The formerly high-achieving student who skips class due to hangovers begins failing key courses and is removed from an honors program or extracurricular team.

These examples highlight how problematic use can quickly shift from occasional substance use to patterns that undermine a young person's well-being, safety, and future opportunities.

Consequences of problematic substance use can impact teens in the following ways, indicating escalating risks: increased risk of disciplinary actions (suspension, expulsion) for substance-related incidents; conflict with parents due to secrecy, lying, or breaking household rules about substance use; increased irritability, mood swings, or emotional outbursts; loss of opportunities (e.g., being removed from sports teams, missing out on scholarships); possible arrest or court involvement for possession, underage drinking, or DUI.

Hazardous/Chaotic Use: Problematic use plus frequent observed risk-taking related to use and developing physical dependence and addiction. Examples are:

- A 17-year-old uses opioid pain pills without a prescription and experiences withdrawal symptoms when they stop using.
- A teen binge drinks (5+ drinks in a short period) multiple times a month, leading to blackouts or risky behavior like driving while intoxicated.
- A college junior uses cocaine regularly to stay awake for work and school, experiencing paranoia and sleep problems.
- A 15-year-old smokes cannabis daily, skipping school and withdrawing from family.

These patterns are often associated with serious and escalating consequences, such as:

- **Physical dependence and withdrawal**: The 17-year-old who misuses opioids begins to experience withdrawal symptoms between uses and may feel unable to stop without help.
- **High-risk behavior and medical emergencies**: The teen who binge drinks experiences blackouts and drives while intoxicated, increasing their risk of injury, arrest, or accidental harm to others.
- **Mental health crises**: The college junior who uses cocaine regularly begins experiencing paranoia, disrupted sleep, and heightened anxiety, which may progress into a mental health crisis.
- **Social isolation and academic failure**: The 15-year-old who smokes cannabis daily begins skipping school, losing contact with friends, and falling behind academically, increasing their risk of dropping out.

Hazardous or chaotic use often signals the need for immediate, intensive intervention. At this stage, the potential for long-term harm – both physical and psychological – is significant, making early engagement and flexible, non-punitive support critical.

Addiction versus physical dependence

Because the term addiction often comes up at the more severe end of the use spectrum, it's important to clarify how it differs from physical dependence and why that distinction matters. The word *addiction* gets used so casually – "addicted to sugar", "addicted to my phone" – that its clinical meaning is often lost. Pop culture and media tend to sensationalize it, reinforcing the idea that any use of an addictive substance automatically equals addiction. But in behavioral health and medicine, *addiction* has a much more specific meaning. According to the DSM-5 (American Psychiatric Association, 2022), addiction – technically referred to as a substance use disorder – is diagnosed based on a pattern of compulsive use, loss of control, craving, and continued use despite functional impairment or psychological distress. It's not defined simply by using a substance, nor by developing tolerance or withdrawal.

The medical definition of *physical dependence* refers to the body's adaptation to a substance over time. With repeated exposure, the brain and nervous system adjust, leading to tolerance (needing more of the substance to achieve the same effect) and withdrawal symptoms when the substance is reduced or stopped. This is a physiological process, not a behavioral one – and it happens even in the absence of addiction. For example, chronic pain patients who take opioids long term almost always develop tolerance and physical dependence. If they suddenly stop their medication, they may experience withdrawal symptoms like sweating, nausea, or agitation. But many of these patients do not exhibit any signs of addiction: they are not using compulsively, not escalating doses inappropriately, and not continuing use despite psychological or social harm. Similarly, post-surgical patients may receive opioids for acute pain and take them exactly as prescribed for a few days. They may still develop a mild tolerance or experience transient withdrawal after stopping – but they don't go on to crave the drug, nor do they seek more. These are classic cases of physical dependence without addiction.

So while addiction may involve physical dependence, the two are not the same. Addiction is a behavioral health diagnosis rooted in compulsive use and psychological dynamics. Physical dependence is a normal, expected biological response to certain medications. Conflating the two – especially in how we label people – does a disservice to both those struggling with SUDs and those managing legitimate medical needs.

To support a deeper understanding of the spectrum of adolescent substance use, we refer you to Exercise 3. This exercise guides you in applying harm reduction principles to real-world counseling scenarios, using the continuum of use as a framework. Through case analysis, role-play, and group reflection, you will practice recognizing different patterns of use and developing developmentally appropriate responses that emphasize safety, engagement, and autonomy.

While the spectrum of use helps us understand *how* often and *how severely* a teen may be using substances, the next step is to consider *how* they're using – and what strategies can support safer, more intentional choices. In the section that follows, we'll explore the Safer Use Continuum as a practical framework for applying harm reduction principles in your work with adolescents.

The Safer Use Continuum

Understanding the specific consequences of substance use along this spectrum enables us to better adopt strategies that minimize harm. The concepts of *safe, moderate*, and *controlled* use are reviewed in Denning and Little's *Over the Influence* (2017) as a framework to help individuals make informed choices about changing their use while balancing risk and personal goals. They recognize that teens will have different goals and capacities for managing substance use while emphasizing strategies to minimize harm rather than impose strict prohibition.

As seen in Table 9.1, we add *safer use* to this gradation of change because it offers more flexibility and another option to minimize immediate risks while keeping communication open. By acknowledging safer use, parents and providers can offer nonjudgmental guidance that promotes informed decision-making and reduces potential harm, rather than pushing teens toward secrecy or riskier behaviors. For teens, however, these phases of change require extra caution, as developing brains are more vulnerable to substance-related harm, and strategies like moderation or controlled use may be harder to maintain due to increased impulsivity and risk-taking tendencies.

The safer use continuum allows for a nonjudgmental and flexible strategy for increasing motivation to change a teen's relationship with substances that meets them where they are and incorporates the harm reduction dictums of "better is better" (Anderson & Smith, 2022) and "small positive steps" (Bigg, 2001). It fosters trust, reduces resistance, and empowers teens to take ownership of their decisions. Small steps leading to small improvements in behavior – the experience of success – increases confidence and hope, which drives the process forward.

Table 9.1 Safer use continuum for adolescents

Category	Definition	Example	Harm Reduction View	Caveats for Teens
SAFE	Choosing not to use substances or engage in any risky behavior; a valid and supported choice within harm reduction.	Total abstinence from substances.	While abstinence is the safest option, harm reduction acknowledges that some individuals may still choose to use substances.	Abstinence is encouraged, as even early experimentation can disrupt brain development and increase the risk of long-term problematic use.
SAFER	Strategies that reduce but do not eliminate harm when using substances. Safer use is relative and depends on context, behaviors, and individual risk factors.	Using a designated driver when drinking. Not mixing substances like alcohol and prescription drugs. Using clean paraphernalia to prevent infections (for substances taken non-orally).	The goal is to minimize immediate risks, such as overdose, impaired judgment, or infections, while recognizing that some level of risk remains	Even with harm reduction strategies, teens have less impulse control and higher risk-taking behaviors. "Safer" does not mean safe, and experimentation can escalate into more frequent use.
MODERATE	Using substances in a limited and regulated manner to reduce potential harm and negative consequences.	Drinking small amounts of alcohol on rare occasions. Using cannabis only in small amounts and infrequently.	Moderate use may be acceptable for adults but is more difficult and presents higher risk for teens due to their developing brains and the potential for misuse.	Teens often struggle with self-regulation, making moderate use difficult to maintain. "Moderate" can be misleading; what seems moderate to one person may still be harmful to another, especially in the period of adolescent development.
CONTROLLED	A structured approach where a person sets strict limits on when, how much, and under what circumstances they use substances to prevent escalation to problematic use.	Only drinking alcohol in social settings and limiting intake to two drinks. Using cannabis only on weekends and in low doses.	This is a realistic goal for some adults but can be a challenge for many.	Teens have a harder time sticking to limits, making controlled use unreliable. The earlier substance use begins, the higher the risk of long-term addiction.

Even a high-achieving child's self-esteem is vulnerable, so it's important to voice appreciation and encouragement for any positive change he or she makes along the way.

We offer Exercise 4 to help illustrate how to better understand and apply the safer use continuum when working with teens, using Table 9.1 as a guide. Before turning to the exercise, it's important to reflect on the tone and intention behind harm reduction responses – because how we engage with teens around substance use often matters just as much as what we say. Harm reduction is not a set of scripts or pre-approved answers – it's a stance. It asks us to let go of assumptions about readiness, compliance, or "doing it right", and instead lean into curiosity, respect, and the belief that small positive steps matter. Across the vignettes in Exercise 4, you'll notice that effective harm reduction responses tend to share a few key features. They begin by *honoring the teen's experience* – not in a way that condones risky behavior, but in a way that validates their autonomy and their reasons for using. Rather than focusing on judgment or control, these responses are built around *open dialogue* and *collaborative risk assessment*, helping teens weigh the impact of their choices in a developmentally sensitive way.

You'll also see that harm reduction approaches tend to *de-shame the conversation*. They avoid moralizing language and instead prioritize education, skill-building, and trust. Even when a teen has clearly made a dangerous choice, like mixing substances or using daily, the harm reduction lens looks for entry points, not endpoints. It's not about "fixing" the behavior on the spot, but about *planting seeds, preserving the relationship, and keeping the door open* for future change.

As you engage with the scenarios, try to resist the urge to steer teens directly toward abstinence or control. Instead, explore what safer use might look like in their world. Ask how their use fits into their goals, how they assess risk, and what support they might need to make a shift – even a small one. Your task isn't to solve the case, but to practice a stance: curious, nonjudgmental, developmentally attuned, and committed to reducing harm – even if that just means making one choice a little safer than the last. Let that orient you as you walk through the vignettes – *not to get it perfect*, but to stretch your comfort with the gray areas and find language that keeps teens engaged, informed, and empowered.

Chapter 10

Adolescent HRT in Practice

Integrated Dynamic Engagement Assessment (IDEA): A Nonlinear and Client-Centered Approach in Working with Adolescents

Traditional addiction treatment models often rely on a diagnostic approach where assessment is used to categorize a client's "problem severity" before prescribing a structured treatment plan. These models assume a linear progression toward abstinence, which usually does not align with how adolescents engage with therapy.

The Multidisciplinary Assessment Profile (MAP), developed by Denning and Little (2012) within HRT, represents a groundbreaking shift in substance use assessment that integrates assessment as an ongoing part of the therapeutic process. Rather than assessing severity and recommending abstinence-based interventions, IDEA adapts the MAP's structure of organizing assessment across multiple life domains to ensure an individually responsive approach to adolescent substance use. IDEA is tailored specifically for working with adolescents by incorporating key adolescent-specific factors, including cognitive development, peer dynamics, family relationships, and emerging identity formation, to create a flexible, client-centered assessment framework.

IDEA, like the MAP, prioritizes engagement, safety, and gradual behavior change over rigid treatment mandates, aiming to develop a nuanced understanding of adolescent substance use within the broader context of overall well-being. IDEA also views assessment as an ongoing, holistic, and interactive process that begins in the very first moments of contact. It considers the adolescent's relationship with substances in relation to their mental health, social environment, cognitive development, and personal strengths – acknowledging complexity rather than pathologizing behavior.

Rooted in the same principles that guide the MAP, IDEA draws from multiple theoretical frameworks to support a comprehensive, flexible, and person-centered approach to assessing adolescent substance use and other risky behaviors. It builds on the foundation of the MAP by adapting it for the unique developmental realities of adolescence. Unlike adults, teens are still forming their identities, developing cognitive and emotional capacities, and navigating complex social environments. IDEA retains MAP's comprehensive structure but integrates developmentally attuned elements that make it more relevant and engaging for young people. It supports a broader understanding of the adolescent's world: their needs, motivations, challenges, and strengths.

As seen in Table 10.1, IDEA adapts the 13 assessment dimensions that Denning and Little (2012) outlined in the MAP and organizes them for adolescents within Zinberg's *Drug, Set, and Setting* framework. This multidimensional structure resists linear or deficit-based approaches to

Table 10.1 Integrated Dynamic Engagement Assessment (IDEA), an adolescent adaptation of the Multidisciplinary Assessment Profile (MAP). Based on Denning & Little (2012), *Practicing Harm Reduction Psychotherapy: An Alternative Approach to Addictions* (2nd ed.). Guilford Press

Domain	Component	Adolescent-Specific Considerations
Drug	Type of substance(s) used	- Substances used (e.g., cannabis, nicotine) - Frequency, quantity, route (e.g., vaping, edibles) - Experimental vs. habitual patterns
	Level of misuse/ dependence	- Impact on daily life (school, sleep, mood) - Perceived control over use - Withdrawal or compulsive patterns?
	Prescribed medications	- Current/past meds (e.g., ADHD, anxiety) - Compliance, misuse, or sharing - Side effects and impact on use
Set	Motivation & expectations for use	- Desired effects (fun, calm, focus, escape) - Emotional, social, or identity-related drivers
	Stated goals	- Preferred changes, substance or otherwise - Willingness vs. external pressure for treatment
	Stage of change	- Precontemplation to maintenance - Awareness and ambivalence about change
	Self-efficacy	- Belief in capacity to change or cope - History of attempts, internal vs. external control
	Treatment history	- Formal/informal help (therapy, school, peers) - What was helpful or harmful
	Psychiatric & medical history	- Diagnoses, symptoms, trauma, health issues - Youth and caregiver perspectives on links to use
	Developmental grid	- Key identity-shaping experiences - School, peer, family, cultural influences
Setting	Setting of use	- Where, when, and with whom use occurs - Social or solitary context; safe vs. risky settings
	Support system	- Family, peers, mentors, community ties - Presence or absence of trusted adults
	Therapist's concerns	- Risks not acknowledged by youth - System pressures (e.g., legal, CPS, school) - Blind spots or safety issues

assessment, providing a non-pathologizing, contextual lens for understanding substance use. Zinberg's framework, initially discussed in the introduction to Part II (*Addressing Substance Use With Harm Reduction Treatment Strategies*), was developed to explain why people use substances in different ways and with varying outcomes. It emphasizes that drug-related consequences are shaped not only by the pharmacological properties of the substance (the *drug*), but also by the individual's internal state (*set*), and the social and environmental context (*setting*) in which use occurs.

Instead of isolating substance use as a standalone problem, the model embeds it within a complex biopsychosocial context – inviting therapists to consider the interplay of pharmacology, internal experience, and environmental influences. This framing supports individualized treatment planning that is adaptive and context-sensitive, rather than prescriptive or narrowly focused on abstinence. In doing so, it operationalizes harm reduction not just as a philosophy, but as a clinical method – one that balances rigor with empathy, and honors autonomy while supporting change.

The drug, set, setting structure also enhances interdisciplinary collaboration by offering a shared language across domains – medical, psychological, social, and beyond. And crucially, it creates room to explore both risks and strengths, allowing for a more complete picture of the young person's life – not just what's going wrong, but what's holding them together.

Referring to Table 10.1, the dimensions are organized into three overarching categories – drug, set, and setting – to align assessment with this ecological and relational understanding of adolescent behavior. Here's how:

- Drug-related dimensions include things like the types of substances used, routes of administration, patterns and frequency of use, and pharmacological effects. This helps clinicians understand the pharmacodynamics involved – but without assuming that all substance use is inherently pathological.
- Set-related dimensions assess the person's psychological and emotional functioning, such as mental health history, coping mechanisms, trauma experiences, and motivational ambivalence. This reflects the "set" of internal variables that influence how and why substances are used.
- Setting-related dimensions explore the client's social world: family dynamics, peer networks, housing, legal involvement, culture, and systems interactions. These highlight the external conditions that shape use, risk, and protective factors.

In work with adolescents who use substances, there's often pressure to act quickly – to assess risk, assign diagnoses, and implement interventions. The IDEA offers an alternative entry point. Rather than rushing toward conclusions or treatment plans, the IDEA invites a pause. It centers relationship-building and curiosity, positioning the assessment process as an opportunity for deeper understanding. With adolescents – especially those who are ambivalent, guarded, or disengaged – this shift in stance can be transformative. The IDEA provides a structure for collaborative exploration, allowing practitioners and teens to reflect together on what substance use means in the context of their broader life: their stressors, relationships, identity, and aspirations.

Through this process, a more nuanced profile begins to emerge. This isn't a static diagnostic picture, but a dynamic, individualized map of the young person's world, highlighting patterns of use, emotional drivers, social context, protective factors, and vulnerabilities. It accounts for the complexity and fluidity of adolescent development, where needs, roles, and risks are constantly shifting. Importantly, it also brings forward strengths and resilience – elements often overlooked in traditional assessments.

Beyond understanding, the IDEA also functions as a practical guide. It helps practitioners identify developmentally appropriate, stage-matched strategies that align with where the adolescent is currently – cognitively, emotionally, and motivationally. Whether a young person is in precontemplation, testing limits, or actively seeking change, the IDEA supports tailored interventions that honor both autonomy and safety. It also promotes coordination across systems – mental health, education, juvenile justice, and family – while keeping the young person's voice and goals at the center. In this way, the IDEA acts as both a framework for engagement and a foundation for integrated, responsive care.

We now take a closer look at interaction of drug, set, and setting as a way to further contextualize the individualized profiles that emerge through the IDEA process, bringing into sharper focus the internal and external conditions that shape how adolescents engage with substances over time.

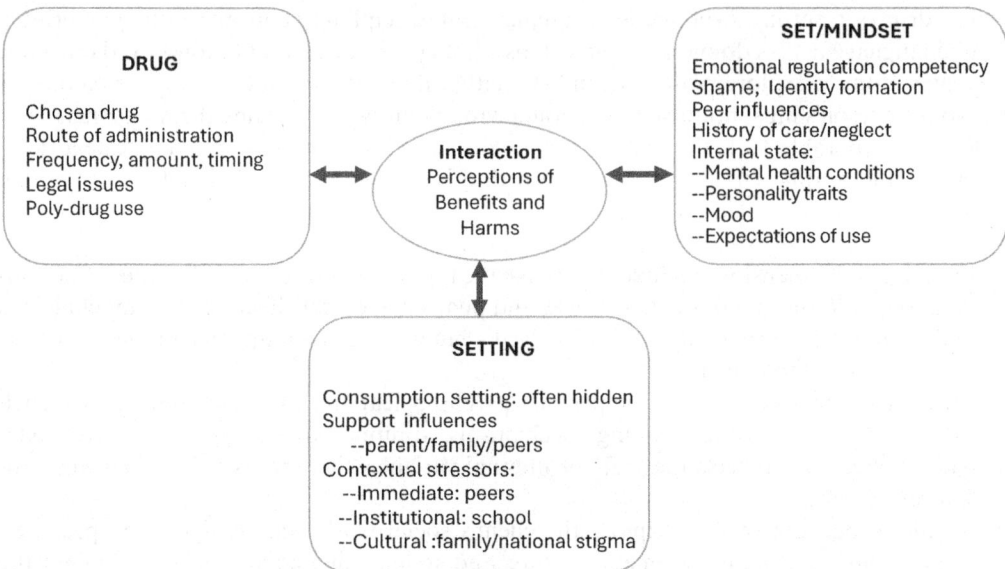

Figure 10.1 Zinberg's drug, set, setting adapted for adolescent development. Based on Denning, P., & Little, J. (2017). *Over the Influence: The Harm Reduction Guide to Controlling Your Drug and Alcohol use* (2nd ed.), p. 101. Guilford Press.

Zinberg's drug, set, and setting: Contextualizing use for tailored interventions

Zinberg's drug, set, and setting framework helps clarify a teen's relationship with substances by examining not just what they use (drug), but also their mindset and motivations (set/mindset), and the social and environmental influences (setting) that shape their experiences. It reframes assessment from stigmatizing substances to a comprehensive exploration of the context surrounding use

In IDEA, it recognizes that adolescent substance use is often driven by peer dynamics, emotional regulation, identity exploration, and access to substances rather than just pharmacological effects. By assessing these interacting factors, IDEA helps clinicians understand the full context of a teen's use, allowing for developmentally appropriate, harm reduction-focused interventions that prioritize engagement, safety, and realistic behavior change. Adolescents' substance use is often shaped by peer dynamics, stressors, and identity exploration rather than entrenched addiction. IDEA ensures that assessment considers social and environmental factors that influence substance use decisions and that interventions become realistic, personalized, and focused on immediate safety and well-being rather than solely on substance elimination.

Drug

A person will have a different relationship with each substance they use. This relationship includes not only the drug's pharmacological properties, but also the meaning the person attaches to it (e.g., "weed helps me chill", or "Adderall keeps me focused"). The dosage and route of administration have important impacts on the outcome of the drug's effect. For example, alcohol products vary significantly in alcohol by volume (ABV): beer and beer-adjacent drinks (5–10% ABV), wines (5–20% ABV), and liquors (15–75% ABV).

Stimulants and opioids can be taken orally, snorted, or injected, each route carrying different risks and effects. Cannabis used for its psychoactive effects can be inhaled (smoking, vaping, dabbing) or orally ingested (edibles, tinctures, capsules). In harm reduction work, this domain also includes the purity and potency of the substance, the risk of contamination, and whether it's used alone or with other drugs (poly-substance use), all of which influence safety and outcomes.

Set (Mindset)

Set refers to a person's internal state, including both stable and variable characteristics that shape their experience when using a substance. This includes personality traits (e.g., glass-half-full versus glass-half-empty worldview), mental health conditions like ADHD, anxiety, or depression, as well as developmental factors (e.g., identity formation, impulsivity in adolescence). Variable aspects of mindset include current mood, sleep, nutrition, and acute stressors, which can change from hour to hour. A critical component of "set" is the person's expectations and intentions: *What do they hope this substance will do for them right now?*

In adolescent work, it's essential to explore how set intersects with:

- Emotional development and regulation capacity
- Shame, identity formation, and peer influence
- Prior experience of care, safety, or systemic neglect

Setting refers to the environment in which substance use takes place. We can understand this better by looking at the different levels of context:

Micro-level: The immediate physical and interpersonal context – where the person is, who they're with, how safe or private the setting is (e.g., using at home, in a car, in secret, with trusted friends, or in unsafe environments).

Mid-level: Institutional contexts that shape the person's daily life and behavior – such as schools, families, foster care systems, the juvenile justice system, and drug treatment programs. These systems can support or undermine safety, especially for marginalized youth.

Macro-level: Broader cultural and structural forces, such as prohibitionist drug policy, stigma, systemic racism, gendered expectations, poverty, and access to healthcare. These factors influence what drugs are available, how people are punished or supported for using them, and how they view themselves as substance users.

Examples of how the model allows for context-sensitive harm reduction planning include:

- If an adolescent uses stimulants to study, interventions may explore academic stressors and alternative study supports before addressing substance use directly.
- If a youth drinks primarily at high-risk parties, interventions may focus on safer drinking strategies or identifying safer social environments.
- If cannabis use is tied to social connection, strategies may explore alternative ways to foster belonging rather than immediately suggesting abstinence.

Importance of the dynamic interaction

Drug, set, and setting are in constant interaction. A stimulant like cocaine, for example, does not produce a uniform effect. An individual may feel energized and socially engaged when using it in a celebratory group setting, yet the same person might experience heightened anxiety or dysphoria when using it alone during a period of emotional distress. The pharmacological properties of the drug remain the same, but the individual's internal state (*set*) and external environment (*setting*) significantly influence the outcome. The same holds true for substances like cannabis: one person may find it calming, while another may become anxious or disoriented, depending on their psychological makeup and the surrounding context. In this way, substance use cannot be understood solely by identifying the drug; it requires attention to the full picture.

This is where the concept of a *substance use profile* becomes especially useful. It serves as a dynamic, individualized map of how, why, when, and under what conditions a person engages with substances. It incorporates behavioral patterns (frequency, quantity, combinations), emotional and psychological drivers (such as coping, identity formation, or social connection), and broader contextual factors (peer influences, family climate, cultural norms, and access). This profile is not static; it evolves over time, shaped by developmental changes, life transitions, and shifting internal and external pressures.

Adopting this perspective is key. It moves us away from assumptions and one-size-fits-all interventions and instead encourages a stance of informed curiosity. What role is the substance playing in this young person's life? What function does it serve, and how do they perceive the risks or benefits? With adolescents in particular, these questions are central. Their substance use patterns are still emerging, and their identities, relationships, and environments are continually in flux. Understanding their unique profile allows us to engage more effectively – meeting them not according to predetermined goals, but in the context of their lived experience.

Within the IDEA framework, the Decisional Balance offers a practical and relational tool for exploring ambivalence – something that's especially common in adolescent substance use. Rather than pushing for immediate change, it invites young people to reflect on both the perceived benefits and the costs of their current behavior. This exploration is not only about identifying risks, but about uncovering the *functions* that substance use serves, whether it's emotional regulation, social belonging, escape, or experimentation. When paired with a needs hierarchy lens, the Decisional Balance becomes even more powerful. It allows practitioners to consider how a teen's use may be tied to unmet or emerging developmental needs, like the need for autonomy, identity, connection, or safety. In this way, the IDEA doesn't just highlight "problem behavior", but helps organize and give meaning to it, grounding it in the broader context of adolescent development.

When used this way, the Decisional Balance becomes less of an intervention technique and more of a tool for insight. It helps clarify internal conflicts that might not yet be fully conscious – conflicts between identity and safety, connection and control, relief and consequence. Framed within the IDEA process, it provides a structure for inquiry, collaboration, and compassionate engagement.

Decisional Balance

Decisional Balance is a structured approach used within MI to help individuals explore the benefits and drawbacks of their behaviors, making it a powerful tool for working with adolescents. Rather than pressuring teens into change, it helps them assess their own motivations, ambivalence, and potential consequences in a way that respects their autonomy. By allowing teens to explore both the benefits and drawbacks of their behavior, it respects their autonomy, helping them arrive at their own conclusions rather than feeling pressured into making decisions they aren't ready for. This approach also reduces defensiveness, acknowledging the reasons behind their substance use – whether for social connection, stress relief, or coping – allowing them to feel understood rather than judged.

We have found that Decisional Balance is a powerful tool that encourages young people to begin sharing about themselves where otherwise they would be reluctant to do so. Beyond fostering open dialogue, Decisional Balance encourages self-reflection, helping teens recognize patterns in their behavior that they may not have consciously considered. Many adolescents have never systematically weighed the impact of their choices, and this process creates space for them to examine both risks and motivations in a non-confrontational way. Even if they aren't ready to stop using substances, the tool supports harm reduction by helping them identify practical ways to minimize risks and make safer choices.

For teens who are unsure about change, Decisional Balance facilitates movement through the stages of change, particularly for those in the contemplation phase. Rather than nudging them toward an endpoint they may not yet be ready for, it provides a structured way to explore their ambivalence and consider whether, when, and how they might want to make adjustments. By meeting teens where they are, Decisional Balance fosters a sense of agency, making it more likely that any changes they choose to make will be meaningful and sustainable. It facilitates a nonjudgmental exploration of the pros and cons of substance use from the adolescent's perspective, helping adolescents self-identify priorities and shape interventions that feel relevant and achievable. It identifies why substance use is appealing (e.g., coping with stress, social bonding), highlights concerns the adolescent may already recognize, and helps them determine what aspects of their use they are willing to modify, rather than imposing external goals.

Elements of decisional balance

The Decisional Balance Matrix consists of four key elements, allowing teens to weigh their choices holistically:

Pros of Using (Why I Do It) – What benefits do they perceive from their substance use or risky behavior (e.g., stress relief, fitting in, feeling more confident)?
Cons of Using (What Problems It Causes) – What negative effects have they noticed (e.g., trouble at home/school, emotional struggles, health concerns)?
Pros of Cutting Back or Stopping (What Could Improve?) – What positive changes might happen if they reduce or change their behavior (e.g., better sleep, improved relationships, less anxiety)?
Cons of Cutting Back or Stopping (What's Hard About Changing?) – What barriers make change difficult (e.g., social pressure, fear of losing friends, not knowing how to cope)?
By mapping out these four areas, teens gain a clearer understanding of their behavior's impact and can begin identifying which aspects they are most motivated to change – helping them form a needs hierarchy to guide intervention strategies.

Decisional balance and needs hierarchy: Understanding motivations & priorities

From this process emerges a needs hierarchy, which structures interventions based on the adolescent's self-identified priorities rather than an externally imposed treatment plan.

Table 10.2 Samantha's Decisional Balance Matrix

Decision	Pros (Reasons to Continue)	Cons (Negative Effects)
Drinking at Parties	Helps me feel more confident Friends expect me to drink Makes me forget stress	I don't remember parts of my night My friend is mad at me I'm worried about unsafe hookups
Cutting Back or Stopping	I'd have better control I wouldn't wake up regretting things Less drama with my friends	Might feel awkward at parties My friends will ask why I'm not drinking I don't know how to handle stress without it

For example, see Table 10.2 for how these priorities can be organized to guide collaborative, developmentally appropriate intervention planning.

- If cannabis use is primarily about managing anxiety, the focus may be on alternative coping skills first, rather than immediate reduction.
- If peer pressure is driving alcohol use, then social skills or boundary-setting interventions take priority.
- If safety concerns arise (e.g., opioid use in high-risk settings), harm reduction strategies are prioritized before behavior change discussions.

Decisional Balance and Needs Hierarchy for Samantha's Risky Behavior

Scenario: **Samantha, a 16-year-old girl, has been drinking heavily at parties, sometimes blackout drinking. She has also been engaging in unsafe sexual activity while intoxicated and recently got into an argument with a close friend about her behavior.**

Determining Samantha's needs hierarchy

Working through this exercise with her therapist, Samantha realizes that her biggest concerns aren't about alcohol itself but about its consequences – blackouts, unsafe situations, and friendships being affected. Instead of pushing for total abstinence, her needs hierarchy could look like this:

1. Reduce risk of blackouts – Strategies: Drink more slowly, alternate drinks with water, set a drink limit.
2. Improve safety in social situations – Strategies: Have a trusted friend at parties, use a "buddy system", avoid situations where she feels pressured.
3. Address stress in healthier ways – Strategies: Find alternative coping skills (e.g., journaling, exercise, talking to a friend).
4. Improve self-confidence without substances – Strategies: Explore self-esteem work, challenge negative self-talk, build social skills for sober interactions.

While the Decisional Balance helps clarify what's at stake for an adolescent – what they value, fear, and hope for – the Stages of Change SOC model offers a way to understand *where* they are in their readiness to act on that awareness. As the final core element of the IDEA process, the SOC model provides a flexible, developmentally attuned framework for pacing interventions to match the young person's current stance toward change.

Stages of Change Model (SOC)

The Stages of Change Model (SOC) helps assess an adolescent's readiness for change and ensures that interventions align with their current motivation and willingness to engage. IDEA integrates the SOC to assess an adolescent's motivational state without pushing premature interventions, ensuring that discussions align with the adolescent's current mindset. Using SOC attuned to youth allows for fluid movement between stages, acknowledging that change is non-linear, especially in adolescence.

Precontemplation – "I don't need to change."

The adolescent does not yet recognize their substance use as concerning. They may be using for social, coping, or exploratory reasons and see no need for change. Therapists focus on trust-building and engagement rather than confrontation.

- Example: A 16-year-old regularly smokes cannabis with friends after school. They say, *"It's not a big deal – everyone does it. It helps me chill."* They don't believe their use has any negative impact and resist discussing change.
- Assessment Approach:
  - Focus on building rapport and exploring their perspective without judgment.
  - Ask open-ended questions: *"What do you like about using? Are there any downsides?"*
  - Introduce Zinberg's drug, set, and setting model to explore relationship with substances and how and why they use.

Contemplation – "Maybe I'll make a change but I'm not sure."

The teen acknowledges some concerns but feels ambivalent about change. They see both benefits and drawbacks of their substance use. Decisional Balance is a valuable tool to assist them explore their motivations.

Example: A 15-year-old drinks at parties and recently got in trouble for sneaking alcohol into a school event. They say, *"Yeah, I guess I could've gotten suspended, but I wasn't even that drunk. I just didn't want to feel left out."*

Assessment Approach:

- Use Decisional Balance: *"What do you enjoy about drinking? Are there times when it hasn't gone well?"*
- Normalize ambivalence: *"It sounds like part of you likes the social aspect, but another part is worried about the consequences."*
- Discuss harm reduction alternatives like setting limits on the amount they drink, avoiding mixing substances, making a plan for getting home safely, or identifying safer social settings where they feel less pressure to use.

Preparation – "I want to change, but I need support."

Adolescents in this stage are thinking seriously about making changes, exploring their options, and starting to make small, practical plans. They may not have it all figured out yet, but they're open to support and actively weighing how to shift their behavior in a way that fits their goals and values.

- Example: A 17-year-old says, *"I've been vaping a lot, and I know it's messing with my lungs. I want to stop, but it's hard because all my friends do it."*
- Assessment Approach:
  - Work together to use the safer use continuum to guide decisions about how to reduce risk in ways that feel realistic and meaningful to them, even if they're not ready to stop using (*"What small steps feel doable?"*).
  - Identify triggers and supports (*"What situations make it harder? Who can help?"*).
  - Offer realistic alternatives (nicotine gum, social strategies for avoiding peer pressure).

Action – "I'm trying to stay on track, but sometimes it's tough."

At this stage, the teen has made meaningful changes and is actively working to maintain them. Challenges, stressors, and occasional lapses are common. Support focuses on sustaining motivation, problem-solving barriers, and reinforcing progress without expecting perfection.

- Example: A 16-year-old who stopped misusing ADHD medication to study for exams uses again during finals week. They say, *"I was doing fine, but then I had a huge test and caved. I feel like I messed everything up."*
- Assessment Approach:
  - Normalize the lapse and affirm that setbacks are part of the change process ("You've been working hard – one slip doesn't erase that progress." Reinforce the idea that the goal is *progress, not perfection*, to reduce self-judgment and build resilience).
  - Explore what was happening before, during, and after the return to use (e.g., academic pressure, emotional state, available supports).
  - Reframe the lapse as a learning opportunity ("What did you learn about what you need during high-stress weeks?").
  - Collaboratively adjust the plan, identifying what might help next time (e.g., more study support, stress management tools, earlier check-ins).

Maintenance/setback prevention – "I've made changes and want to keep them going."

After sustaining change over time, the focus shifts to reinforcement and setback prevention. The adolescent has sustained changes over time and is building confidence in their ability to manage risk and avoid return to old patterns.

Example: A 15-year-old who hasn't smoked cannabis in several months says, *"I still think about it sometimes, but I don't want to mess up how far I've come."*

Assessment Approach:

- Identify what's working and highlight the teen's own strategies for success.
- Explore ongoing vulnerabilities and co-develop a plan for high-risk situations.
- Revisit motivation and ensure goals still align with current values.
- Support continued identity development that reinforces the change.

Bringing It All Together

The following case example brings together all core elements of the IDEA framework – offering a practical, harm-reduction-informed lens for understanding and responding to the complex realities of adolescent substance use, emotional distress, and developmental needs.

Scenario: Brianna is a 16-year-old girl referred by a community mental health clinic due to school truancy, family conflict, and concerns about cannabis and alcohol use. She lives with her aunt and younger cousin following her mother's incarceration, and her relationship with her aunt is strained but caring. Brianna came to treatment voluntarily, though hesitantly, saying her aunt hoped "someone would actually listen without judging". She presents with housing instability, school disengagement, and growing ambivalence about her substance use.

1. *Substance Use History*
   Overview:
   Brianna began using cannabis at 14 and now uses it almost daily. She also drinks alcohol occasionally at parties. She describes weed as something that "keeps her calm", helps her sleep, and makes "everything quiet". Most often she uses alone, especially after school or during moments of stress or conflict. There is no indication of physical dependence, but cannabis has become her primary coping strategy.
   Drug, Set, and Setting:

   - Drug: Cannabis, used regularly, mostly smoked. Occasional alcohol use.
   - Set: Internal state marked by anxiety, emotional overload, and chronic fatigue.
   - Setting: After school, often alone, occasionally with friends in public parks or unsupervised settings. Use is more frequent when she feels overwhelmed, angry, or hopeless.

   Harm Reduction Perspective:

   - Normalize the use as an attempt to regulate distress, not simply "bad behavior".
   - Explore connections between use and unmet needs for safety, autonomy, and soothing.
   - Discuss ways to reduce harm (e.g., using in safer contexts, moderating amount, not mixing with alcohol).
   - Offer science-based psychoeducation resources about how cannabis may affect memory, sleep cycles, and anxiety over time.

2. *Psychiatric and Emotional Functioning*
   Overview:
   Brianna describes persistent sadness, irritability, and moments of emotional shutdown. She denies active suicidality but admits to thoughts like, "I wish I could just disappear." She shows signs of panic and hyperarousal under pressure. She avoids vulnerability, stating, "talking to people just makes it worse".
   IDEA/SOC:

   - Presenting in contemplation around understanding her emotional distress; not ready to explore deeper trauma but recognizes that "something's off".
   - IDEA process reveals trauma-related symptoms likely tied to family disruption, housing instability, and emotional isolation.

Harm Reduction Perspective:

- Prioritize consistency and trust-building; avoid pushing for disclosure too early.
- Frame symptoms as understandable responses to chronic stress.
- Introduce non-pathologizing language (e.g., "your nervous system is working hard to protect you").
- Offer low-barrier regulation tools (e.g., music, movement, grounding exercises) that she can try on her terms.

3. *Cognitive and Behavioral Functioning*
Overview:
Brianna is articulate and insightful but reports trouble with focus, memory, and organization, especially when stressed or after using cannabis. Teachers describe her as intelligent but disengaged. She skips class and often appears exhausted or detached when she does attend.

Decisional Balance:

- Pros of use: Reduces overthinking, helps her "turn off" emotionally, makes school feel more bearable.
- Cons: Fatigue, zoning out in class, conflict at home, awareness that it may be affecting her ability to focus.

Harm Reduction Perspective:

- Validate her struggles as impacts of trauma, not laziness or defiance.
- Co-create manageable academic goals (e.g., "Try attending 3 out of 5 days").
- Explore organizational tools that feel age-appropriate and empowering (e.g., use of phone reminders instead of paper planners).
- Expand definitions of success – what else makes her feel competent?

4. *Health and Medical*
Overview:
Brianna is disconnected from medical care. She avoids clinics due to past negative experiences and fears of being judged. She has difficulty sleeping, often skips meals, and reports chronic fatigue. She has untreated dental issues and limited food access at home.

Harm Reduction Perspective:

- Explore what kind of provider feels safest to her (e.g., someone younger, female, nonjudgmental).
- Normalize avoidance of systems that have previously failed or harmed her.
- Set achievable steps (e.g., "Would you be open to texting with a clinic instead of calling?").
- Connect her with food pantries, teen clinics, or mobile care units once some trust is established.

5. *Family and Social Relationships*
Overview:
Brianna lives with her aunt and cousin in a small apartment. The relationship with her aunt is tense; her aunt tries to set limits but struggles with consistency. Brianna feels both judged and cared for. Her mother is incarcerated and contact is sporadic. Brianna has a small social circle, but keeps emotional distance.

IDEA/Needs Hierarchy:

- Strong themes of attachment disruption, role confusion, and emotional isolation.

- Substance use appears tied to a desire for emotional independence and a break from caregiving stress.

Harm Reduction Perspective:

- Acknowledge complexity in her family dynamics without idealizing "support".
- Help her define boundaries in relationships – what feels draining versus what feels safe.
- Explore safe practices in romantic/sexual relationships without shame or assumption.
- Validate her loyalty and ambivalence around caregiving roles.

6. *School and Academic Functioning*
Overview:
Brianna is in 11th grade but at risk of not graduating on time. She is behind in multiple classes, with inconsistent attendance. She expresses shame about her performance but resists help. Teachers vary in how they perceive her; some see her potential, others write her off as oppositional.

SOC/Decisional Balance:

- In preparation around re-engaging with school in some form.
- Open to alternative options but wary of failure and being labeled.

Harm Reduction Perspective:

- Collaborate on minimal, achievable goals (e.g., "Let's focus on passing two core classes this term.")
- Explore alt pathways (online, GED, work-based programs) without judgment.
- Identify one supportive adult at school who can serve as a point of stability.
- Reinforce non-academic sources of self-worth – art, caregiving, humor, problem-solving.

7. *Legal and System Involvement*
Overview:
No active charges, but Brianna has had school-based warnings for cannabis use and truancy. She has a strong mistrust of authority and fears being criminalized. Her mother's incarceration deeply shapes her perception of the justice system.

IDEA/SOC:

- In precontemplation about formal system engagement but aware of risk.
- Motivated by self-protection more than fear of punishment.

Harm Reduction Perspective:

- Validate her fear and mistrust as adaptive – not resistant or oppositional.
- Collaborate on safety plans (e.g., knowing rights, avoiding use in public).
- Emphasize intrinsic motivation – "What helps you feel in control?" rather than relying on fear of consequences.
- Hold space for conversations about systemic injustice and her lived experience.

Clinical considerations for treatment planning

- Brianna is navigating intersecting challenges: trauma, economic hardship, racialized systems, disrupted attachment, and stigma.
- Substance use functions as a primary regulatory tool, especially for emotional distress and identity protection.

- Therapy must begin with relationship-building and emotional safety. Pacing and collaboration are essential.
- Caregiver support may need to focus on shifting from control to attunement and capacity-building.
- Community-based resources (food, housing, education, peer support) are not peripheral; they are central to sustainable change.
- Therapeutic stance: non-expert, collaborative, culturally responsive, and flexible. Focus on "with", not "for" or "to".

Having explored the IDEA framework as a foundation for engaging adolescents through individualized, developmentally responsive assessment, we now turn to the evidence-based treatment modalities that often complement this approach. While IDEA helps us understand *who* the young person is and *how* substance use fits into their world, approaches like Harm Reduction Therapy (HRT), Motivational Interviewing (MI), Cognitive Behavioral Therapy (CBT), and Dialectical Behavior Therapy (DBT) offer concrete strategies for supporting change. Each of these modalities can be adapted to meet teens where they are – honoring ambivalence, centering agency, and building the skills needed to navigate distress, relationships, and risk with greater awareness and capacity.

Motivational Interviewing

Motivational Interviewing (MI) is a client-centered, directive, counseling approach designed to enhance intrinsic motivation for behavior change by resolving ambivalence. Developed by Miller and Rollnick (1991, 2012), MI is rooted in collaboration, evocation and autonomy, making it particularly effective for adolescents, who often resist authority-driven interventions. Evocation refers to the process of drawing out a client's own motivations, values, and strengths rather than imposing external advice or solutions. The therapist is directive in this sense–instead of telling the client why they should change, evocation encourages the client to articulate their own reasons for change, making it more personally meaningful and sustainable.

By balancing client-centered conversation with gentle direction, MI is highly effective when working with adolescents (Dean et al., 2016; Jensen et al., 2011), helping young people explore their substance use, consider potential risks, and identify personal goals for change, without imposing external expectations. A key component of MI is exploring ambivalence, helping teens reflect on both the positive and negative aspects of their substance use. Questions such as, *"What do you like about using? What are some things you don't like?"* invite open discussion, allowing the young person to consider their own motivations rather than being told what to do. From there, counselors can elicit change talk by asking questions like, *"If you decided to cut back, what might that look like?"* – helping adolescents imagine realistic adjustments to their behavior on their own terms. MI also emphasizes reframing risk, shifting the conversation from judgment to practical safety strategies, such as *"What are some ways you could make your use safer?"* Finally, MI helps build self-efficacy, reinforcing a young person's ability to make meaningful changes by highlighting past successes: *"You've already made some changes – what helped you do that?"*

The effectiveness of MI in harm reduction lies in its core principles. Expressing empathy through reflective listening validates an adolescent's experiences and reduces defensiveness. Developing discrepancy helps them recognize the gap between their current behaviors and future goals, enhancing motivation for change. Instead of challenging resistance, MI rolls with it, avoiding direct confrontation and working with the adolescent's perspective rather than against it. Supporting self-efficacy reinforces the idea that they are capable of making changes, no matter how small. Instead of demanding abstinence, MI enhances motivation for incremental change, encouraging safer behaviors that are meaningful and sustainable. It also integrates well with the Stages of Change model, allowing providers to tailor interventions to whether an adolescent is precontemplative, contemplative, or ready for action. Because it is non-coercive and collaborative, it improves engagement and retention, increasing the likelihood that adolescents will stay in treatment and explore their options.

The following case example offers an overview of how MI can be applied in practice, particularly with a mandated client who is initially resistant to change. See Exercise 5 for a structured opportunity to engage more deeply with MI through role play, reflection, and applied skill-building.

Case Example Demonstrating MI: A 19-year-old college sophomore arrested for DUI

Background: Sara, a 19-year-old college sophomore, was arrested for DUI after leaving a party. She was mandated to attend substance use treatment as part of a diversion program. Sara reports that "everyone drinks in college", denies having a serious problem, and expresses frustration about being forced into treatment. However, she acknowledges feeling embarrassed about the arrest and worried about potential long-term consequences.

Since Sara is mandated to treatment and initially resistant, the therapist takes a nonjudgmental, client-centered approach that fosters engagement and relational safety as a foundation, rather than emphasizing abstinence.

1. *Establishing Rapport and Expressing Empathy*

Therapist: *"It sounds like you feel frustrated about being here and don't think drinking is a big issue for you. That makes sense – getting mandated to treatment when you don't feel you need it can be annoying. I appreciate you showing up and being open to talking about it."*

- Why? This validates Sara's feelings and reduces defensiveness, setting the stage for collaboration.

2. *Exploring Ambivalence Using Decisional Balance*

Therapist: *"I hear that drinking is a normal part of your college experience. Can we explore that a little? What do you like about drinking? And what are some things you don't like, especially after the DUI?"*

- Why? This helps Sara reflect on both the benefits and drawbacks of her drinking without feeling judged.

Possible Responses from Sara:

- Pros of drinking: "It's fun, helps me relax, and makes socializing easier."
- Cons of drinking: "Getting arrested sucked. I don't want to lose my license or mess up my future."

By guiding Sara to express concerns on her own, the therapist avoids confrontation and fosters self-motivation.

3. *Developing Discrepancy and Eliciting Change Talk*

Therapist: *"You mentioned that drinking helps you have fun, but the DUI put your license and future at risk. On a scale of 1 to 10, how important is it for you to avoid another DUI?"*

If Sara rates it highly (e.g., 8/10), the therapist can build on that:
Therapist: *"That's pretty high. What makes it an 8 instead of a 4?"*
If Sara rates it low (e.g., 3/10), the therapist avoids arguing and instead asks:
Therapist: *"What would need to happen for that number to go up?"*

- Why? This reinforces Sara's own reasons for change rather than imposing external pressure.

4. *Identifying Harm Reduction Strategies*

Since abstinence is not the goal, the therapist collaborates with Sara on practical strategies to reduce harm:

- Safer drinking habits: Setting a drink limit, alternating alcohol with water, or tracking consumption.
- Reducing risk of DUI: Using rideshares, a designated driver, or staying at a friend's place.
- Recognizing risky patterns: Identifying situations where they are more likely to overdrink.

Therapist: *"What are some things you'd be willing to do differently to make sure you don't end up in this situation again?"*

- Why? This allows Sara to take ownership of her behavior rather than feeling lectured.

5. *Supporting Self-Efficacy and Strengthening Commitment*

If Sara expresses interest in change, the therapist reinforces her ability to follow through.
Therapist: *"It sounds like you're thinking about making some changes. You've already handled tough situations before. What's helped you follow through when you set a goal?"*
If Sara remains resistant, the therapist keeps the door open:
Therapist: *"You're the expert on your life. My role isn't to tell you what to do but to help you figure out what works for you. If you ever want to talk more about this, I'm here."*

- Why? This avoids pressure, making Sara more likely to engage in future sessions.

This case example illustrates how MI can be effectively applied with a mandated client who is initially resistant to treatment. Sara, a 19-year-old college student arrested for DUI, enters therapy believing her drinking is typical for someone her age and resents being forced into treatment. The therapist adopts a nonjudgmental, person-centered stance focused on rapport-building, empathy, and engagement rather than confrontation or imposing abstinence.

Key takeaways for counseling practice include: validating client resistance to reduce defensiveness; exploring ambivalence using decisional balance; developing discrepancy through reflective questioning; and eliciting change talk without pressure. Importantly, the therapist supports harm reduction by collaboratively identifying realistic strategies to minimize risk, such as using rideshares or setting drinking limits. Throughout, the therapist reinforces self-efficacy and autonomy, keeping the door open for future engagement. This case highlights how MI can meet clients where they are while still promoting insight, motivation, and safer choices.

Cognitive-Behavioral Therapy

Cognitive Behavioral Therapy (CBT) is one of the most well-established, evidence-based approaches for treating substance use among adolescents. Hogue et al. (2014) and Tanner-Smith et al. (2013) confirmed in meta-analyses that CBT – particularly when tailored to adolescents' developmental needs – can significantly reduce substance use frequency and related distress. These findings are especially robust when CBT is combined with motivational interviewing and CBT family-based therapy.

CBT's strength lies in its ability to help adolescents understand and manage the internal and external triggers that contribute to substance use or other risky behaviors. When teens use substances in response to emotional discomfort – anxiety, shame, boredom, loneliness – or in specific environments that make use feel expected or unavoidable, CBT helps them "map" these situations by understanding the relationship between their thoughts, emotions, and behaviors – essentially "connecting the dots" – to bring subconscious patterns into conscious awareness. They can notice their patterns of behavior, and begin to experiment with alternative ways of responding. For example, an adolescent who smokes cannabis every day after school to "chill out" may, through therapy, identify that this urge often follows a spike in tension or irritability after being in an overstimulating school environment. CBT helps them examine the automatic thought – "If I don't smoke, I won't be able to relax" – and challenge it by introducing new coping options such as listening to music, journaling, or using movement to release energy. The goal is not to take away the substance use but to create new options, so the young person feels more in control of how they respond to discomfort.

In the authors' clinical experience, CBT is especially effective with adolescents when it includes developmentally attuned, non-shaming education about the brain's stress response. Teaching teens how their amygdala triggers the fight, flight, or freeze response – and how this temporarily limits the availability of the prefrontal cortex (which manages impulse control and decision-making) – helps them understand why they may feel emotionally flooded or act impulsively in moments of stress. By educating clients about this neurobiological pattern, CBT normalizes their reactivity and reduces shame. It reframes substance use as a learned way to manage overwhelming states, rather than a failure of willpower. Through consistent practice – like identifying emotional cues early, pausing before acting, or applying grounding techniques – adolescents strengthen the neural pathways involved in regulation and choice.

Another essential component of CBT is building metacognition: the ability to observe one's own thoughts and urges without being ruled by them. For young people, this is a powerful shift. They begin to understand that they don't have to act on every craving, and that they can choose how to respond to discomfort, stress, or peer influence. Tools like thought logs, trigger mapping, and functional analysis help make their internal experience more visible and manageable. In this way, CBT becomes a tool not just for behavior change, but for self-understanding and empowerment. Within a harm reduction model, it supports adolescents in becoming more curious about their patterns, more compassionate with themselves, and more equipped to make choices that reflect their evolving values. Whether they're trying to reduce their use, avoid high-risk situations, or simply feel more in control, CBT offers practical skills grounded in respect for their autonomy and developmental stage.

Dialectical Behavior Therapy

Dialectical Behavior Therapy (DBT) is an evidence-based treatment developed by Marsha Linehan (2015) to address chronic emotion dysregulation, self-harm, and suicidal behaviors, particularly in individuals with borderline personality disorder. Grounded in cognitive-behavioral theory, DBT integrates principles of dialectics and mindfulness, drawing from both Western psychology and Eastern contemplative practices. Its central dialectic – balancing acceptance with change – enables clients to validate their current experiences while also developing new, more effective coping strategies.

Recognizing the need for adolescent-specific adaptations, Rathus and Miller (2002) developed Dialectical Behavior Therapy for Adolescents (DBT-A) in collaboration with Linehan. DBT-A modifies the original model to meet developmental needs and involves caregivers in multi-family skills groups. DBT-A acknowledges the critical role of family systems in adolescent treatment and provides concrete, developmentally appropriate tools for navigating peer conflict, impulsivity, and identity development. A growing body of research supports DBT's effectiveness with adolescent substance users. Groves and Van Sciver (2022), in a systematic review of DBT for adolescents with substance use disorders, found that DBT led to reductions in substance use frequency, emotional reactivity, and treatment dropout. These findings reinforce DBT's relevance as a harm reduction-aligned intervention that not only targets substance use but also addresses the emotional and relational contexts in which it occurs. With its emphasis on skill-building, validation, and behavioral flexibility, DBT offers a responsive and evidence-based framework for supporting both adolescents and adults in reducing harm and building lives that feel more manageable – and more worth living.

Chapter 11

Trauma-Informed Care

Trauma and addiction are deeply interconnected, with a growing body of research and clinical experience showing that substance use often emerges as a strategy to manage the emotional, psychological, and physiological effects of trauma. Rather than being purely recreational or self-destructive, many individuals – especially those with histories of abuse, neglect, systemic oppression, or complex developmental trauma – turn to substances to regulate overwhelming feelings, numb distress, or create a sense of control and safety. In this context, effective treatment must acknowledge the protective role substances can play while supporting clients in developing new ways of coping.

Building on Denning and Little's harm reduction therapy model, which has been central to this discussion, this section broadens the lens by examining other influential contributors who position trauma as central to understanding and treating substance use. Their models offer valuable tools for engaging clients with empathy, flexibility, and respect – particularly when substance use serves as a means of coping with emotional distress or trauma. We will then return to Denning and Little to take a closer look at how their model integrates trauma-informed care within a harm reduction framework, with particular attention to how their approach can be effectively adapted to meet the developmental and relational needs of adolescents.

Andrew Tatarsky's work, as mentioned earlier in Chapter 6, has played a key role in shaping a harm reduction approach that is clinically rigorous while also being deeply attuned to the emotional realities of clients, offering a thoughtful and compassionate way to understand substance use as a meaningful response to pain, not just a problem to eliminate. His Integrative Harm Reduction Psychotherapy (IHRP) also centers trauma in its understanding of substance use, but with a slightly different clinical emphasis than Denning and Little. Tatarsky focuses on how trauma shapes the emotional, cognitive, and relational meanings of substance use, particularly in clients with complex histories of invalidation, shame, or neglect. His model views substance use as a form of self-regulation and protection – a way to manage intolerable affect, unmet attachment needs, or fragmented identity. Unlike traditional psychodynamic models that view addiction as regression or resistance, IHRP treats it as a meaningful, even adaptive, coping strategy.

IHRP addresses trauma through a process of collaborative inquiry that allows clients to gradually develop insight into their patterns, emotional drivers, and unmet needs. Rather than imposing abstinence, Tatarsky works to increase curiosity, awareness, and internal coherence, helping clients connect current behaviors to past experiences, often revealing early relational trauma or chronic misattunement. Clients are invited to reflect on the emotional logic of their substance use, not to pathologize it, but to gain power over it. As trust builds, therapy may include affect-regulation strategies, mindfulness, and cognitive restructuring, but always within a flexible, trauma-sensitive frame. Trauma is not a target to be "processed" in a linear way – it is unfolded organically through exploration of the self in relation to others and to substance use.

While IHRP was originally developed for adults, its emphasis on meeting clients where they are, reducing shame, and exploring the emotional and relational meaning of substance use makes it adaptable for adolescents. The author has adapted IHRP for use in clinical work with adolescents by translating its reflective, client-driven framework into more accessible, practical interventions. This includes using language and metaphors that resonate with teens – connecting substance use to familiar challenges like school stress, peer pressure, and identity struggles – rather than relying on abstract psychodynamic ideas that may not yet be developmentally accessible. Session structure is also modified to reflect how teens naturally engage. While adults may benefit from longer, open-ended conversations, adolescents often respond better to shorter, more active sessions that incorporate structured dialogue, creative tools like journaling, drawing, or music, and hands-on skills practice tied to their current lived experience. To support insight and behavior change, the adaptation includes weaving in emotion regulation and executive functioning strategies, drawing from Dialectical Behavior Therapy (DBT), Cognitive Behavior Therapy (CBT), and mindfulness approaches, helping teens bridge the gap between recognizing patterns and learning to pause or self-regulate in real time.

Because adolescent substance use is often deeply connected to social context and peer belonging, sessions also include space to explore friendships, group dynamics, and how substances are used as a tool for fitting in, coping, or asserting autonomy. We have discussed previously how important family engagement is, so collateral therapy sessions with parents (with consent by the teen client) focus on psychoeducation, communication strategies, and aligning support around the teen's goals without compromising their autonomy. CRAFT approaches are often integrated into the treatment. Finally, goal setting is adapted to be flexible and teen-centered, often broken down into smaller, time-limited steps that reflect what feels possible and meaningful to the adolescent. These adaptations preserve the heart of IHRP – meeting clients where they are – while making it responsive to the developmental realities of adolescence.

Lisa Najavits (2022) is a leading psychologist and researcher in the field of trauma and addiction, best known for developing the widely used treatment model *Seeking Safety*. Her work focuses on treating individuals with co-occurring posttraumatic stress disorder (PTSD) and substance use disorders and challenges the idea that trauma must be fully processed before addressing addiction. Instead, she offers integrated, flexible, and client-centered approaches that prioritize safety, stabilization, and practical coping skills. More recently, Najavits developed Creating Change (2022), a past-focused, structured treatment for those who are ready to engage more directly with trauma content. This model complements *Seeking Safety* by offering a next step for clients who have stabilized and want to explore deeper trauma work.

Throughout her work, Najavits emphasizes compassion, empowerment, and flexibility, making her models especially suitable for clients with complex trauma histories and co-occurring disorders. Her contributions have been instrumental in shaping trauma-informed, integrated care in both research and practice. To illustrate how *Seeking Safety* can be effectively integrated within a harm reduction framework for adolescents, the following vignette presents a clinical example of working with a teenager who continues to use substances while engaging in therapy.

Vignette: Tara, Age 16 – Integrating *Seeking Safety* with Harm Reduction Therapy

Tara, a 16-year-old high school student, was referred to therapy by her school counselor after repeated cannabis use on campus, failing grades, and signs of depression. She lives with her aunt following a history of emotional neglect and exposure to domestic violence in her early childhood. Tara insists she's "not ready to stop smoking", describing cannabis as her "only way to calm down" when overwhelmed. Rather than pushing abstinence, the therapist begins with a harm reduction stance, building rapport and validating Tara's coping strategies as survival-based responses to trauma.

Using *Seeking Safety*, the therapist introduces core topics such as "Safety", "When Substances Control You", and "Grounding". These sessions help Tara recognize the connection between her substance use, emotional dysregulation, and unresolved trauma, without requiring her to process traumatic memories directly. She especially connects with the concept of "Honesty" – realizing she's been hiding pain and fear behind a tough exterior. Over time, Tara begins experimenting with alternative coping skills, such as journaling and sensory grounding exercises, and she sets a personal goal to reduce school-day cannabis use to avoid further suspensions.

Like HRT, *Seeking Safety* accepts that clients may continue using substances while engaging in treatment. Both models prioritize emotional safety, skill-building, and self-determination, making them highly compatible in adolescent work. While HRT provides a flexible, relational foundation rooted in client-defined goals, *Seeking Safety* offers a structured, trauma-informed toolkit that can support stabilization and empowerment – even when abstinence isn't the goal.

Bessel van der Kolk is a psychiatrist and trauma researcher whose work has been instrumental in advancing our understanding of how trauma affects the body and brain. Best known for his book *The Body Keeps the Score* (2014), van der Kolk emphasizes that trauma is not just a psychological experience but a deeply physiological one, often encoded in the nervous system and expressed through chronic dysregulation, dissociation, and somatic symptoms. His work highlights how trauma can impair the brain's ability to regulate emotion, particularly through disrupted connections between the amygdala, prefrontal cortex, and insula, leading many trauma survivors to live in a chronic state of hypervigilance or emotional numbness.

Rather than focusing solely on talk therapy, van der Kolk advocates for bottom-up, body-based treatments that target the neurobiological imprint of trauma. These include practices such as yoga, Eye Movement Desensitization and Reprocessing (EMDR), sensorimotor psychotherapy, neurofeedback, and theater/movement-based therapies, all aimed at helping individuals reestablish a sense of bodily safety and self-regulation. His approach is especially relevant for work with adolescents, whose nervous systems are still developing and are highly sensitive to environmental stressors.

While van der Kolk does not explicitly identify with harm reduction, his emphasis on respecting the adaptive function of trauma responses, and avoiding retraumatization by working at the client's pace, aligns with the core values of harm reduction therapy. His framework is particularly useful when working with youth who struggle with emotional regulation, dissociation, or substance use as a form of somatic relief. For clinicians, van der Kolk's work reinforces the need to engage the body, brain, and relational context of trauma, and to move beyond purely cognitive interventions in the treatment of complex trauma and its behavioral manifestations.

Van der Kolk's work offers powerful insights into the neurobiological and somatic impact of trauma, making it highly relevant for teens struggling with emotional dysregulation and body-based symptoms; however, some of his theories and recommended interventions (e.g., yoga, neurofeedback) lack consistent empirical validation in adolescent populations and may require careful adaptation to be developmentally appropriate and evidence-informed.

After reviewing other models that offer different perspectives into working with trauma, we now return to Denning and Little's HRT model to more closely examine how their approach addresses trauma as a core component of substance use. They frame trauma as deeply intertwined with – and often driving – substance use patterns. They define trauma broadly, including not only acute or chronic interpersonal trauma (e.g., abuse, neglect), but also systemic and developmental traumas, such as racism, poverty, incarceration, or institutional betrayal. Substance use is often described by clients as their most effective – or only – strategy for managing emotional overwhelm, numbness, or fear. They treat trauma as central to therapy but emphasize that effective trauma treatment must begin with safety, stabilization, and trust, especially for clients with complex trauma histories. And rather than pushing for disclosure or deep processing early on, their model focuses first on reducing shame, supporting emotional regulation, and creating a therapeutic environment where clients feel seen and accepted – even while continuing to use substances. This brief vignette illustrates this:

> Maria, age 15, was referred to therapy by her school counselor after multiple suspensions for vaping cannabis and frequent absences. She lives with her grandmother after being removed from her mother's care due to years of neglect and exposure to domestic violence. Since the removal, Maria has bounced between relatives and short-term placements, and she rarely talks about her past. At intake, she says, "I don't need therapy – I just want people to leave me alone."
>
> Rather than confronting her use or pressing for a trauma narrative, the therapist takes a harm reduction stance, focusing on creating safety and building rapport. They ask about what *Maria likes* about cannabis, when she uses it, and what it helps her manage. Maria eventually shares that smoking helps her sleep and feel less angry. The therapist gently reflects how hard it must be to carry that much anger and exhaustion, and validates her strategy as one way she's learned to survive. Over time, they explore ways Maria can tell when she's "about to shut down", and experiment with grounding techniques she can use in class or at home.
>
> As trust builds, Maria begins to describe feeling like no one listens to her unless she's in trouble, and that school feels like "a place where I'm already expected to fail". Rather than interpreting her cannabis use as resistance, the therapist frames it as a response to overwhelming stress and emotional disconnection. With the therapist's support, Maria starts identifying safer spaces and people in her life and begins to imagine other ways to cope, even if she's not ready, or interested, in quitting.

This vignette demonstrates the core principles of Denning and Little's approach, particularly their emphasis on safety, stabilization, and respect for the client's coping strategies. It prioritizes relationships, emotional safety, and the client's autonomy, allowing a teen like Maria to build skills and insight without needing to disclose or stop using right away. Her substance use is not ignored but understood in context – as a survival tool shaped by trauma, not as a failure of character or motivation.

The Role of Attachment in Trauma

Attachment theory, originally developed by John Bowlby (1988), provides a foundational understanding of how early relational experiences shape emotional development, coping strategies, and long-term psychological well-being. Bowlby proposed that infants are biologically predisposed to form attachments with caregivers to ensure survival, particularly during times of distress. When these needs are met with consistency and emotional attunement, children typically develop secure attachment styles, which support emotional regulation and resilience. However, when caregiving is neglectful, inconsistent, or frightening, children may develop insecure or disorganized attachment patterns, which are associated with emotional dysregulation, impaired trust, and increased vulnerability to maladaptive coping strategies later in life.

Mary Ainsworth's (1978) research further elaborated on Bowlby's theory by identifying distinct attachment patterns through her *Strange Situation* studies and introducing the concept of the caregiver as a "secure base". These patterns influence how individuals respond to stress and seek out comfort – dynamics that remain highly relevant during adolescence, a developmental stage marked by increasing autonomy, emotional intensity, and identity exploration. For teens with histories of disrupted attachment, substance use may emerge as a way to self-soothe or regulate overwhelming emotions, particularly when supportive relational frameworks are absent or unreliable.

In this context, Denning and Little's HRT model offers a particularly relevant application of attachment theory. In *Practicing Harm Reduction Psychotherapy* (2012), they describe how early attachment disruptions – whether due to trauma, loss, neglect, or systemic harm – leave individuals without the internal scaffolding needed to manage distress, seek help effectively, or build trusting relationships. As a result, substances often become substitute attachment objects – predictable sources of relief, comfort, or control in a world that otherwise feels unsafe or emotionally barren.

Denning and Little emphasize that substance use is not simply a pathological behavior, but a deeply embedded relational and emotional adaptation, particularly for those with attachment wounds. Their model places the therapeutic relationship at the center of healing, viewing it as a reparative experience where clients – especially adolescents – can begin to experience emotional safety, consistency, and respect. Rather than pushing for abstinence or emotional disclosure early in treatment, HRT prioritizes stabilization, trust-building, and emotional regulation, in line with what Bowlby described as the core conditions for secure attachment.

Importantly, Denning and Little broaden the attachment lens to include not only interpersonal trauma, but also systemic and developmental traumas – such as racism, poverty, incarceration, and institutional betrayal – that further compound attachment injuries. For adolescents navigating these overlapping layers of harm, substance use may serve as both coping and resistance. Within a harm reduction framework, attachment-informed care means meeting teens where they are, validating the function of their substance use, and offering relationships that don't retraumatize or demand change as a prerequisite for care.

Understanding attachment theory and its role in trauma offers valuable insights into how early relational experiences shape emotional development and coping, allowing clinicians to respond to substance use not simply as a behavior to change, but as a reflection of unmet needs for safety, regulation, and connection.

Chapter 12

Working with Parents

This chapter introduces Community Reinforcement and Family Training (CRAFT), an evidence-based, skills-oriented approach for helping parents support a teen who is using substances. The chapter explores how CRAFT can be adapted for work with adolescents across developmental stages and levels of risk. Through case examples and clinical teaching points, you'll see how this model helps shift family dynamics from conflict to collaboration, even when the teen is ambivalent about change. To further support families, the chapter concludes with a curated list of science-based resources, support groups, and tools specifically designed for parents.

CRAFT (Community Reinforcement and Family Training)

Robert J. Meyers' innovative development of *Community Reinforcement and Family Training* (CRAFT) in the mid-1990s marked a paradigm shift in the field of substance use treatment, particularly in how families and concerned significant others (CSOs) are supported (Smith & Meyers, 2023). As the only empirically supported approach specifically designed for concerned significant others (CSOs) of people using substances, CRAFT introduced a compassionate, evidence-based alternative to confrontational models. Grounded in behavioral principles, CRAFT focuses on positive reinforcement, effective communication, and family empowerment to support both the individual using substances and the broader family system. It aligns closely with harm reduction philosophy by meeting people where they are and promoting small, meaningful steps toward change without imposing rigid expectations or moral judgments.

Unlike the more widely known Johnson Institute Intervention (JII), which is structured around a single, high-stakes confrontation, CRAFT relies on non-confrontational strategies that emphasize collaboration and incremental progress. In a typical Johnson Intervention, family members plan a surprise meeting to confront the person using substances with ultimatums and emotional appeals, aiming to pressure them into immediate treatment. While widely practiced, this model can backfire and lead to defensiveness, ruptured relationships, and resistance, especially when the person is not ready to accept help. CRAFT, by contrast, teaches CSOs how to gradually shift the environment around their loved one to encourage treatment readiness. This includes learning how to reinforce healthy behavior, reduce enabling patterns, and re-engage in activities that bring meaning and self-respect back to the family system (Meyers & Smith, 2023).

The effectiveness of CRAFT was demonstrated in a 2002 randomized clinical trial by Meyers, Miller, Smith, and Tonigan, which compared CRAFT to both the Johnson

Intervention and Al-Anon/Nar-Anon Facilitation (ANF) (Meyers et al., 2002). The study found that 64% of substance users whose family members were trained in CRAFT entered treatment within three months, compared to only 23% in the JII group and 13% in the ANF group. Beyond increasing treatment engagement, CRAFT also improved the emotional well-being of family members. Participants reported reductions in depression, anxiety, and anger, along with increased feelings of empowerment and improved relationship quality, even when their loved one did not enter treatment.

CRAFT's behavioral roots draw heavily on principles of operant conditioning and skills-based learning, which make it particularly compatible with authoritative parenting practices, as discussed in Chapter 9. For example, family members are trained to reinforce behaviors that are incompatible with substance use – such as attending work or spending time with family – by offering praise and connection, thereby increasing the likelihood of those behaviors recurring. Conversely, they are encouraged to disengage and withdraw rewards during periods of substance use, employing the principle of extinction rather than punishment. This strategy helps reduce the reinforcement of substance-using behavior while avoiding confrontational interactions.

Communication is another core component of CRAFT. Family members learn to express themselves using nonjudgmental, empathetic, and assertive language, often through the use of "I" statements. Instead of saying, "You're always drinking", a family member might say, "I feel worried when I see you drinking a lot." This shift fosters openness and reduces defensiveness, making space for more effective and respectful dialogue.

CRAFT also introduces families to Functional Analysis, a structured method for understanding substance use patterns. By identifying antecedents (what happens before use), the behavior itself, and its consequences, families can better understand what maintains the use, and how to shift those contingencies to promote change. This helps relatives move away from unintentional reinforcement or rescuing behaviors and instead support natural consequences (e.g., allowing someone to face the outcome of missing work due to drinking) without adding shame or punitive responses.

Importantly, CRAFT places strong emphasis on the health and well-being of family members themselves. It teaches self-care, boundary setting, and the importance of maintaining personal interests and independence. This not only reduces burnout but also models healthier relational dynamics and improves the family's overall resilience, regardless of whether the loved one chooses to enter treatment. To illustrate how these principles unfold in real time, the following case study demonstrates the application of CRAFT within a family navigating a loved one's ongoing substance use and ambivalence about treatment.

After outlining the types of interventions used in CRAFT, we now turn to two case examples that show how it can be integrated into work with adolescents across different developmental stages. These examples reflect the model's flexibility across different developmental needs and levels of risk – one involving a college student engaged in excessive drinking, and the other focused on a younger adolescent with acute mental health concerns. Together, they highlight how CRAFT strategies can support harm reduction, build family engagement, and promote change in the kinds of situations counselors often encounter in practice.

The first case we review in the sidebar illustrates how CRAFT principles can be applied in work with parents who are increasingly concerned about their son Alex's drinking and related behaviors:

Case Example: The Rodriguez Family and Their Son, Alex

The Rodriguez family has been struggling with their 19-year-old son, Alex, who has been drinking heavily and frequently missing his college classes. His parents, Maria and David, are worried but unsure how to help without pushing him away.

Functional analysis: Identifying patterns

Through Functional Analysis, Maria and David work with a counselor to identify the antecedents, behavior, and consequences of Alex's drinking.

- Antecedents: Stress from school, conflict at home, peer influence.
- Behavior: Drinking alone or with friends, staying out late, missing class.
- Consequences: Temporary relief from stress, peer acceptance, but also poor grades and tension at home.

They recognize that Alex's drinking is often triggered by academic pressure and that when he drinks, they unknowingly accommodate his behavior by making excuses for him with professors and helping him catch up on missed assignments.

Communication skills and nonjudgmental language

Instead of confronting Alex with accusations like, "You're ruining your future with drinking", they practice nonjudgmental, empathetic, and clear communication using "I" statements.

- Maria tells Alex, "I feel really worried when I see you drinking a lot because I care about your health and future."
- David adds, "I'd love to spend more time together when you're feeling good, like when we went hiking last weekend."

This shift in language makes Alex feel less defensive and more open to conversation.

Positive reinforcement for sober behaviors

Using operant conditioning, Maria and David begin noticing and reinforcing behaviors incompatible with drinking.

- When Alex wakes up early for class, they express appreciation: "I know school is stressful, but I really admire how you're sticking with it."
- When he chooses to stay in and watch a movie with them instead of going out drinking, they order his favorite takeout as a reward.

Over time, this increases the likelihood that Alex will engage in sober activities.

Extinction: Withdrawing attention from substance use

Previously, when Alex came home drunk, Maria would lecture him, and David would argue, which often escalated into fights. With CRAFT's extinction approach, they now disengage without confrontation.

- If Alex comes home intoxicated, they calmly say goodnight and remove themselves from the situation, denying him the attention and engagement he might expect.
- The next morning, rather than cleaning up after him or excusing his behavior, they allow him to experience the natural consequences of his actions – waking up late and struggling through the day.

Allowing natural consequences without punishment

Maria and David decide not to cover for Alex when he misses class due to drinking. When he asks them to call his professor with an excuse, they gently say, "I know this is tough, but it's important to take responsibility for your commitments." When Alex sees that his parents are no longer shielding him from consequences – but also not shaming or punishing him – he begins to reconsider his choices.

Self-care and boundary-setting for the family

Maria and David also recognize the importance of prioritizing their own well-being. They set firm boundaries, ensuring they continue their hobbies and social lives without being consumed by Alex's drinking. Maria starts attending a yoga class, and David reconnects with old friends. This shift not only improves their mental health but also models healthy self-care for Alex.

This case demonstrates how CRAFT can support steady, relational progress, even when change is incremental. As Alex begins to drink less and take greater responsibility, the Martinez family gains a renewed sense of connection and confidence. With education and support, they learn to trust their instincts and apply CRAFT strategies in ways that feel authentic and sustainable. While families can begin using these techniques on their own, working with a trained CRAFT-trained therapist can deepen the process by offering tailored feedback and helping parents stay grounded through inevitable setbacks.

The next case example shifts to an earlier stage of adolescence and a more acute clinical presentation. It explores how CRAFT can be adapted when substance use is entangled with significant mental health concerns and heightened family distress, highlighting the model's flexibility across developmental and diagnostic complexity.

Case Example: Engagement at the Margins of Care – Supporting a High-Risk Adolescent (Bryan, Age 14)

This case explores how CRAFT strategies were applied with the parents of Bryan, a 14-year-old adolescent presenting with daily cannabis use, emotional distress, and escalating conflict at home. Resistant to formal treatment and experiencing waves of suicidal ideation, Bryan's situation highlights the complex intersection of mental health risk, substance use, and adolescent autonomy. The case demonstrates how harm reduction, when combined with parental support and emotional regulation, can provide a path forward – even in the absence of a fully engaged client.

Background: Bryan, a 14-year-old freshman in high school, was referred to counseling by his parents due to daily cannabis use, including before school. Despite being in gifted classes and excelling as a drummer, he has struggled with ADHD and academic frustration. He had a history of inconsistent use of prescribed stimulant medication, citing discomfort with its effects. His parents, in a stable and loving marriage, discovered his diary detailing sadness, hopelessness, and suicidal ideation, leading to significant distress. Bryan refused individual treatment or psychiatric evaluation, and his behavior did not meet involuntary commitment criteria. Attempts to set limits on his cannabis use or enforce curfews often escalated into intense conflicts, including belligerence, threats toward parents, and suicidal threats.

Family Therapy Using CRAFT

Since Bryan initially refused treatment, his parents engaged in therapy without him, utilizing CRAFT (Community Reinforcement and Family Training) to:

- Improve communication and reduce power struggles.
- Set healthier boundaries around substance use and behavior.
- Balance safety concerns with maintaining a positive relationship.

Teaching point: The role of CRAFT in harm reduction

CRAFT helps parents reinforce positive behaviors and reduce unhelpful reactions (e.g., catastrophizing, authoritarian approaches).

- Encouraging parental self-care and emotional regulation reduces their tendency to react out of fear.
- Avoiding punitive responses helps maintain connection, preventing further alienation.

Social Environment and Risky Behaviors

Bryan had a diverse friend group and a supportive girlfriend. He was passionate about skateboarding and worked as an instructor at a summer camp. However, he engaged in risky skateboarding behaviors (e.g., in prohibited areas), leading to a serious ankle injury. His school later contacted his parents about suspected drug dealing, alleging he sold cannabis to a student who was hospitalized.

Teaching point: Managing risky behavior without escalation

- Balancing safety and autonomy: Adolescents will take risks; punitive interventions (e.g., school suspensions, legal involvement) may push them further into risky environments.
- Parental responses matter: Parents must decide when to intervene and when to allow natural consequences.
- Counselor's role: Supporting parents in reducing punitive responses while still holding boundaries.

Mental Health and Crisis Situations

Bryan occasionally called in distress, reporting obsessive self-harm thoughts, feeling overwhelmed and scared. While he was sometimes acutely suicidal, most instances involved intense distress and self-harm urges rather than active suicidal planning. He agreed to try an antidepressant medication, though he expressed skepticism about its effectiveness, wanting immediate relief rather than long-term solutions.

Teaching point: Crisis management in a harm reduction framework

- Distinguishing between acute versus chronic risk:
  - Does he have a clear plan and intent to die, or is he seeking relief from distress?
  - Over-reliance on hospitalization can undermine trust and reinforce avoidance of therapy.
- Safety planning versus control:
  - Standard safety plans are often ineffective in moments of distress.
  - "Being with" rather than "fixing" helps adolescents feel supported rather than pathologized.
- Parental reactions impact crisis outcomes:
  - Bryan's mother catastrophized, which escalated his distress.
  - Using CRAFT, she learned to stay calm, validate, and provide support without reinforcing crises.

Ethical Dilemmas: Privacy and Autonomy

Bryan remained resistant to ongoing therapy but would reach out in emergencies. His lack of engagement in regular treatment raised challenges regarding confidentiality and parental involvement.

Teaching point: Managing privacy and risk in adolescent treatment

- Ethical gray areas:
  - What to disclose to parents versus what to keep private to maintain trust.
  - Balancing harm reduction with duty to protect.

- Therapeutic alliance is key:
  - Pushing too hard on formal treatment can lead to dropout.
  - Flexible engagement allows Bryan to feel in control of his support.

Balanced Approach: Navigating Substance Use and Autonomy

Bryan had been using cannabis since age 12 and had experimented with LSD and mushrooms.

Teaching point: Applying a harm reduction lens to substance use

- Non-judgmental curiosity: Instead of focusing on eliminating cannabis use, explore:
  - What does he like about it?
  - How does it help him cope?
  - What are the downsides?

- Encouraging self-reflection:
  - How does cannabis impact his goals (e.g., music, relationships, school)?
  - Can he explore other coping strategies?

- Empowerment through choice:
  - Shifting from control-based approaches to guiding informed decision-making.

Outcomes and Growth Areas

Progress Over Time: His parents were reminded that Bryan's problems developed over several years and it will take some time to see some improvements. They were educated about how progress in treatment is not linear but follows a path of "two steps forward, one step back" (Denning & Little, 2017; Marlatt & Donovan, 2005).

- Parental dynamics improved:
  - Father moved away from authoritarian tactics, learning to engage more constructively.
  - Mother learned to regulate emotional responses, supporting Bryan without panic.

- Bryan remained resistant to formal therapy but continued crisis check-ins.
- Substance use persisted but became more reflective:
  - He recognized some negative impacts and began experimenting with moderation.
- Self-harm thoughts continued but with better coping strategies:
  - He learned to reach out for support rather than acting impulsively.

Remaining Challenges

- How to further engage Bryan without pressure.
- How to manage parental expectations while respecting Bryan's autonomy.
- How to continue balancing risk versus trust in counseling.

Bryan's case raises several critical themes relevant to work with high-risk adolescents: the limits of control-based approaches, the need for nuanced safety planning, and the emotional toll on caregivers navigating fear and uncertainty. Through the use of CRAFT, Bryan's parents were able to reduce reactivity, strengthen their connection with him, and begin responding more effectively to crises. While Bryan remained resistant to formal therapy, moments of contact, especially during times of distress, offered openings for reflection and gradual change. This case illustrates the importance of flexibility, trust-building, and realistic pacing when working with youth who are not yet ready for traditional treatment but still need meaningful support.

This next case illustrates how harm reduction principles can be applied in the context of a family supporting a teen with layered mental health and substance use concerns, where multiple systems and stressors are at play.

Case example: Jason, a college student with co-occurring disorders: Bipolar disorder, substance misuse, and trauma

Background

Jason is a 20-year-old college junior diagnosed with bipolar disorder in high school. He has a history of inconsistent medication adherence, excessive alcohol and cannabis use, and multiple treatment attempts (residential, intensive outpatient therapy (IOP), individual outpatient therapy). His father died when he was 8 years old, and he has been raised by his mother, Karen. He has experienced up to a year of stability, but his current setback includes failing out of school and exhibiting severe manic symptoms, including:

- Staying awake for multiple days at a time.
- Grandiose and impulsive behavior (spent $2,000 in one weekend on musical equipment he doesn't know how to use).
- Psychotic thinking (accuses best friend of trying to "steal his ideas" and cut off contact).
- Increased substance use (binge drinking, frequent cannabis use, possible stimulant use).

The college mental health crisis center has now called his mother, requesting that Jason return home due to his instability. Karen is overwhelmed and scared, unsure how to support Jason.

The harm reduction therapist focus is on balancing:

1. Supporting Karen through her fear and distress.
2. Engaging Jason while maintaining trust.
3. Addressing the need for psychiatric re-evaluation.
4. Exploring the impact of substance use on mood instability.
5. Understanding how unresolved trauma influences Jason's crisis.
6. Connecting Karen to support (e.g., NAMI Family Support Groups).

Teaching Point #1: Acknowledging Karen's fear and connecting her to support
Challenge: Karen is terrified and feels powerless watching Jason unravel. She needs support and education on how to respond effectively. Validate her fears and connect to National Alliance on Mental Illness Support Groups (NAMI, n.d.)

- Therapist to Karen: *"Watching Jason go through this must be terrifying. You are not alone. There are support groups for parents who are in your exact situation."*
- Therapist to Karen: *"Have you heard of the National Alliance on Mental Illness (NAMI)? They have support groups for parents dealing with severe mental illness in their kids."*
- Benefits of a NAMI Family Support Group for Karen:
  - Provides connection with other parents facing similar struggles.
  - Teaches effective ways to communicate with a loved one in mania.
  - Helps Karen avoid burnout by building her own support network.
  - Therapist provides Karen with NAMI meeting links and encourages her to join.
- Also suggest Karen obtain an individual therapist for additional support.

Teaching Point #2: Managing grandiosity and impulsivity
Challenge: Addressing grandiosity directly can escalate defensiveness and damage therapeutic rapport. Instead, use reflective listening and curiosity to slow down impulsivity.

- Therapist to Jason: *"It sounds like you're feeling really confident and full of ideas right now. What's one step you'd take to make sure they actually work?"*
- Therapist to Karen: *"Rather than challenging Jason's beliefs, help him slow down by asking practical questions about his plans."*
- Avoid head-on confrontation of unrealistic ideas.
- Encourage Jason to take small, practical steps to slow impulsivity.
- Validate his excitement while introducing realistic concerns.

Teaching Point #3: Responding to delusions and paranoia
Challenge: Arguing against delusions increases distress. Instead, focus on Jason's emotions rather than the content of his beliefs.

- Therapist to Jason: *"That sounds really intense. It must be stressful feeling like people are watching you. What's been helping you feel safe?"*
- Therapist to Karen: *"Avoid arguing with Jason's delusions. Instead, acknowledge his emotions and focus on immediate safety."*
- Do not attempt to "correct" delusions. Instead, validate his distress.

- Shift the focus to coping strategies and immediate needs rather than reinforcing paranoia.
- Monitor for escalating paranoia that may require crisis intervention.

Teaching Point #4: Addressing the impact of substance use on mania
Challenge: Many clients do not recognize the link between substance use and worsening mania. Helping them track their experiences can increase insight over time.

- Therapist to Jason: *"You've mentioned that cannabis helps you relax. Have you noticed any times where it's made things feel worse?"*
- Therapist to Karen: *"The goal isn't to get Jason to stop using everything overnight. It's to help him recognize what's making his symptoms worse so he can make more informed choices."*
- Help Jason explore patterns between his substance use and mood instability.
- Introduce harm reduction strategies (e.g., limiting cannabis during manic episodes).
- Encourage small changes rather than all-or-nothing thinking.

Teaching Point #5. Exploring the role of trauma in the current crisis
Challenge: Early trauma can resurface in times of stress, fueling mania and paranoia. Addressing this without overwhelming the client is key.

- Therapist to Jason: *"When things feel really out of control, does anything ever remind you of when you lost your dad?"*
- Therapist to Karen: *"Sometimes, past losses can resurface during times of stress. Do you think Jason's struggles now connect to what he went through as a kid?"*
- Acknowledge that Jason's trauma may be fueling his distress.
- Introduce connections gently without pushing Jason to process trauma prematurely.
- Help Karen recognize trauma responses rather than viewing Jason's behavior as defiant.

Teaching Point #6: Navigating the need for a psychiatric re-evaluation
Challenge: Jason is likely to resist psychiatric intervention unless he feels he has control over the process.

- Therapist to Jason: *"It seems like things have been moving really fast for you lately. Have you noticed any changes in how your mind is working?"*
- Therapist to Karen: *"We may need to work together to get Jason into a psychiatric appointment. That could mean finding a time when he's more open to it or framing it in a way that doesn't feel like a loss of control for him."*
- Frame medication adjustments as a "fine-tuning" process, not a loss of autonomy.
- Encourage Jason to take ownership of his care by involving him in discussions about his treatment.
- If inpatient care becomes necessary, explore harm reduction-oriented hospital alternatives rather than traditional coercive approaches.

Takeaways for Harm Reduction Therapists
This case highlights the interplay between bipolar disorder, trauma, substance use, and family dynamics, reinforcing harm reduction, engagement, and safety planning as key intervention strategies:

1. Manic behaviors can be risky and impulsive. Help slow Jason down without dismissing his reality.
2. Psychotic symptoms require careful navigation. Avoid direct contradiction, instead offer grounding techniques.
3. Jason's trauma may be resurfacing. His fear of losing control and abandonment issues may be at play.
4. Outpatient therapy is limited in acute mania. Focus on containment and stabilization, not deep emotional work.
5. Karen needs support too. Connecting her to NAMI family groups helps prevent burnout.
6. Medication discussions should be collaborative. Avoid ultimatums and instead explore adjustments that Jason can agree to.
7. Balance autonomy and safety in crisis planning. Preemptive harm reduction should be prioritized before forced hospitalization.

When working with a client like Jason, it's important to maintain a therapeutic mindset that prioritizes connection over control. His manic state, paranoia, and impulsivity make it unlikely that he will comply with treatment demands if he feels pressured or coerced. Rather than trying to force stability, the goal is to engage him in a way that makes him feel heard and respected. By prioritizing collaboration over confrontation, Jason is more likely to trust the therapeutic process and consider support options that feel manageable to him.

In moments of crisis, it is essential to remember that small steps matter. Rather than immediately focusing on long-term treatment goals or complete behavioral change, addressing Jason's most basic needs – sleep, nutrition, and immediate safety – comes first. Helping him regain some level of physical stability may reduce his emotional intensity and increase his ability to engage in bigger-picture decisions about medication, therapy, and substance use.

At the same time, parental support is as critical as client support. When parents are exhausted, overwhelmed, and operating from a place of fear, they may unintentionally escalate conflict or reinforce power struggles. Ensuring that Karen has her own emotional support, practical guidance, and community resources (such as NAMI Family Support Groups) will better equip her to navigate Jason's crises without burning out or reacting in ways that drive further disengagement. A well-supported parent leads to a better-supported client, creating a stronger foundation for long-term stability and harm reduction.

Case example: Matt, high school senior

This case example of Matt illustrates how early engagement, parent involvement, harm reduction, and motivational strategies can support a teen navigating depression, insomnia, and daily cannabis use.:

Matt was a month from his 18th birthday, during the summer before his senior year of high school, when his father called for a consultation about Matt's cannabis use. Matt's father reported that he and Matt's mother were extremely worried about their son's seemingly depressed mood, insomnia, underachieving in school and lack of motivation about making a decision about his future. They had lost the ability to trust him since he had been lying about his cannabis use.

Three months prior to the initial call they grounded him and limited his cell phone use after they caught him smoking cannabis in the house and driving after smoking, following repeated warnings to him to stop smoking. They feared that his cannabis use was a gateway to other drug use. They doubted that they could persuade him to come for help and that if he did, he would not participate. Their belief that he would need to hit bottom before responding to any offered help contributed to them feeling helpless. They had previously called another addiction treatment provider, who refused to see them because Matt was not ready to make a change and advised that forcing him to come to treatment would be fruitless. The therapist encouraged Matt's parents to tell him that they had made a decision to consult a professional for some guidance, to invite Matt to the consultation, but that it was his choice to attend or not.

Matt agreed to attend the initial session. The therapist was pleasantly surprised by this, but this was not unusual when the parents adjust to meet their teen where they are at. The harm reduction collaborative approach was discussed with him, and Matt would decide what goals to work on if he chose to continue working with the therapist. At that point, Matt agreed to continue. Once the therapist educated him about the relationship we have with substances, Matt was motivated to talk about his life. He loved playing basketball, hanging out with friends, and earning money from his part-time job. Academics came easy for him, requiring little studying to maintain good grades. He was protective of his younger sister and kind to his grandparents.

But he was furious at his parents for grounding him and for demanding abstinence from cannabis use before he would be trusted enough to be granted more independence. He admitted being depressed since middle school; not being able to see his friends now made him feel more depressed. He went on to share that he was extremely overwhelmed about not knowing what he wanted to do after high school. He said his struggle with insomnia began at the start of high school. He felt unable to share any of these worries with his parents because they thought smoking cannabis was the cause of all of his problems.

They explored his relationship with cannabis (along with the other substances he used regularly, alcohol and nicotine) including the drug, set, and setting for each substance and weighed the pros and cons of his cannabis use. They discussed the spectrum of substance use and whether safe, safer, moderate, or controlled use might be appropriate for him. He admitted smoking cannabis almost daily for two years. He denied that it was a problem for him; he actually saw it as a benefit because smoking cannabis had become the only way he could fall asleep. He shared being frightened to reduce his cannabis use because he didn't think he would be able to fall asleep. He was open to thinking about changing his use when the therapist reassured him that insomnia is a common problem and that they could discuss ways he can improve his sleep in future sessions.

When regaining parental trust was discussed as an issue, he, like most teens, agreed to attend at least one family session. He also agreed to involve his parents more consistently after being reassured that the content of his individual therapy would remain private, and that the therapist would maintain an atmosphere of emotional safety during family sessions. He also agreed to have his parents involved in family sessions after he was reassured of the privacy of the content of his therapy session and with the intention of the therapist maintaining an atmosphere of emotional safety in the session.

Matt shared his treatment goals with his parents and asked them to join him for family sessions. His parents were very relieved that Matt was able to share his feelings of depression and anxiety. His father admitted battling depression and insomnia throughout his life and was able to support Matt mood's difficulties. His mother admitted smoking cannabis a lot in her youth and said that she eventually stopped smoking as her life responsibilities increased. Once Matt's parents were able to view his use as self-medication for his anxiety, depression and insomnia, they were more willing to look at alternative approaches for intervening with Matt.

The therapist used the opportunity to educate them about cannabis and the myth of gateway drugs, and referred them to science-based resources.

Matt used some of his time in therapy to explore career options. After speaking with a military recruiter who came to a career day at his school, he felt confident that the military would be a realistic option for him to get training in his mechanical interests, develop motivation and independence, and to help his parents pay for college when he was ready to enroll. The requirement of the military for Matt to be drug-free at the time of his enrollment evaluation, together with his excitement about his newfound sense of purpose, motivated him to decide to "end his relationship" with cannabis for now. The content of Matt's treatment then focused on his developing healthy strategies and tools to reduce anxiety and improve his mood. He was able to fairly easily stop using and his treatment ended once he was accepted into the military.

Teaching Points

- Challenging the "Hitting Bottom" Myth
  - Many parents, influenced by War on Drug narratives, believe that their child must hit "rock bottom" before they will change. This belief often delays intervention and increases risks (e.g., overdose, legal consequences, mental health deterioration).
  - HRT challenges this myth by engaging individuals where they are, focusing on incremental progress rather than crisis-driven intervention.
  - In Matt's case, early intervention was possible because his parents sought help before his substance use moved further down the use spectrum and experience more consequences. CRAFT approaches empower parents with skills to increase likelihood for their family members to engage in treatment.
- The Problem with "Tough Love" and Zero-Tolerance Approaches
  - Fear and misinformation contribute to parents' discovery of substance use with extreme measures such as grounding, removing privileges, and demanding abstinence. These zero-tolerance policies create a rigid, threat-driven dynamic that heightens family anxiety and pushes teens toward secrecy, often increasing risk.
  - Matt's anger and reluctance to communicate with his parents were direct consequences of their "lockdown" response. CRAFT helped parents shift from punishment to understanding, rebuilding trust and opened space for positive change.
- Dynamic Integrated Assessment: Engaging Teens in Their Own Process
  - Traditional models see assessment as a preliminary step, but HRT treats it as an ongoing process that begins to motivate self-reflection and change.
  - People use substances for reasons. The therapist engaged him in a discussion of his relationship with cannabis with Matt believing that cannabis helped him sleep.
  - Educating Matt about adolescent brain development and the risks of daily cannabis use allowed him to make more informed decisions.
- Using the Stages of Change to Support Readiness for Change
  - Precontemplation: Matt initially didn't see his cannabis use as a problem.
  - Contemplation: Through discussion, he became open to considering change.
  - Preparation: Realizing military enrollment required abstinence, he saw a personal reason to quit.
  - Action and Maintenance: He developed alternative coping strategies for anxiety and sleep, allowing him to sustain changes.
  - Rather than demanding immediate abstinence, HRT support individuals at different points in the Stages of Change, increasing the likelihood of longer-term success.

- Science-Based Education as a Tool for Engagement
  - Providing parents with research-backed information fosters collaboration rather than conflict, increasing their willingness to support harm reduction strategies.
  - The therapist helped Matt's parents shift from seeing his use as a moral failing to understanding it as self-medication for anxiety, depression, and insomnia.
- Risk Management and Small Positive Steps
  - Small, achievable steps create confidence and momentum for change. Zero-tolerance policies prevent this by allowing no flexibility.
  - MI helped Matt acknowledge his fears about reducing cannabis use and work toward alternative solutions for insomnia.
  - HRT and CRAFT with parents emphasized reinforcing safer choices and small improvements rather than demanding immediate, total abstinence.
- Meeting Teens Where They're At
  - Adolescents are naturally resistant to therapy if they feel judged or controlled.
  - HRT and CRAFT prioritize listening, collaboration, and autonomy, allowing teens to engage at their own pace.
  - Matt's case shows that when given autonomy in his treatment, he was willing to engage and ultimately make meaningful changes.
- Engaging and Educating Parents in the Process
  - Parent involvement is essential, but must be handled with care and empathy.
  - Educating families on adolescent brain development and harm reduction can shift responses from punishment to partnership.
  - Resistance is common. Matt's parents initially saw harm reduction as enabling, but became supportive after learning about its evidence base.
  - A teen's refusal to engage in treatment isn't a dead end. It's an opportunity to help parents shift their approach, build connection, and influence change through their own actions and responses.

For Direct Work with Adolescents: An Overview of A-CRA

Although this book focuses primarily on caregiver-centered interventions like CRAFT, we also want to introduce you to a related model, A-CRA, that applies similar principles directly in work with adolescents. A-CRA is an evidence-based behavioral intervention designed for adolescents and young adults (ages 12–24) experiencing SUDs. A-CRA shares foundational elements with CRAFT, including the emphasis on positive reinforcement, communication skills, and functional analysis of substance use. However, A-CRA is delivered directly to the young person (rather than to family members alone) and includes caregiver involvement through separate and joint sessions to support family communication and structure.

Specific elements of A-CRA include functional analysis of substance use and pro-social behavior, where adolescents identify triggers and consequences of their actions, helping them understand what drives their substance use. The program also includes skills training in areas such as problem-solving, communication, refusal skills, emotion regulation, and relapse prevention. Adolescents are supported in developing a daily activity schedule to increase engagement in meaningful, substance-free activities. Parallel sessions for caregivers focus on improving parent-teen communication, positive reinforcement techniques, and strategies for reducing conflict. Joint sessions then bring families together to practice these skills in a supportive, structured environment. Sessions are highly individualized and delivered in-home or in outpatient settings, making the model flexible and accessible.

Research, including findings from SAMHSA's Assertive Adolescent and Family Treatment (AAFT) initiative (Godley et al., 2010) and a comparative outcomes study on adolescents and emerging adults (Smith et al., 2011), have shown that A-CRA is effective in reducing substance use, improving treatment retention, and supporting long-term well-being.

Mutual Help

Despite the growing recognition of harm reduction as a viable and evidence-based approach to adolescent substance use, there remains a notable lack of support groups specifically designed for parents within this framework. Most widely available family resources – such as Al-Anon and Nar-Anon – are grounded in 12-step philosophy and abstinence-only models. These programs have helped many families and can be meaningful sources of support; harm reduction respects their value while also recognizing that different paths to well-being work for different people. Harm reduction seeks to expand the range of options, especially for families seeking a more collaborative, flexible, and developmentally attuned approach.

One important alternative is the SMART Recovery Friends & Family program (SMART Recovery, n.d.), which draws on principles from CBT and CRAFT to offer a nonjudgmental, skills-based approach to improving communication, reducing enabling behaviors, and reinforcing positive change – without requiring immediate abstinence. Developed by clinical psychologist Tom Horvath, SMART Recovery represents one of the most well-established non-12-step mutual help models and aligns closely with harm reduction values.

For more information about this and other resources for parents and families refer to Appendix B.

Chapter 13

Exercises

Exercise 1: Principles of Harm Reduction

For this exercise, place each concept of harm reduction below in the context of working with adolescents. For each concept, answer the following questions:

1. How does this concept relate to society's view of adolescents and adolescent behavior?
2. What are some examples of how a service provider could explore this concept when working with an adolescent client?
3. What are the biggest barriers towards adopting this concept in the context of adolescent and family therapy?

1. **Accepts that substance use is a part of society. Believes that working to reduce the harms associated with use is more beneficial than ignoring or condemning use.**
2. **Acknowledges that substance use is complicated and multi-faceted. Recognizes that there is a spectrum of use, from abstinence to experimentation to regular use, and that there are steps that can be taken to reduce the chance of harm across the spectrum of use.**
3. **Focuses on quality of life as an indicator of success rather than the ability to maintain abstinence.**
4. **Promotes policies and programs rooted in nonjudgment that provide and encourage respect for participants and communities.**
5. **Includes the voices of people who do or have used substances in the creation of policies and programs.**
6. **Supports that people who use drugs (PWUD) have the power to act as agents of change and safety in their own lives and the lives of those in their communities.**
7. **Understands the role that racism, sexism, poverty, and trauma play in both access to services and vulnerability to hazardous substance use.**
8. **Recognizes that substance use can lead to very real harms both at a personal and societal level.**

Exercise 2: Cannabis and Harm Reduction in an Age of Legalization

Now cannabis is legal in states across the country, the conversations we have with teens about use must shift as well. While cannabis was formerly lumped into the category of "illegal" drugs, now the message around cannabis use is more similar to alcohol. While we do not endorse the use of cannabis or alcohol for adolescents, the approach of "never" use, may be adjusted to that of "delay" use. So, how does harm reduction fit into this? In the following exercise, we are providing some scenarios that may be addressed by counselors in a school, or by adolescent and family therapists in the field. For each scenario, think about how you would approach it as a social service professional and from a harm reduction perspective. For each one, answer the following questions:

1. What are the immediate threats of harm (if any)?
2. What are the intermediate threats of harm (if any)?
3. What are the long-term threats of harm (if any)?
4. In these scenarios, what are the risks associated with consuming cannabis?
5. Given how you have answered 1–4, what recommendation would you make to this teen regarding the scenario presented?

Scenario 1: The party

There is a teen (they are 16) you have been seeing in your role as school counselor. They were referred to you because they were having trouble concentrating in class. After meeting with them, you discover that they are distracted because their dad lost his job and there has been stress at home. There is no previous evidence of substance use, other than a few beers here and there at a party, and no evidence of substance use at home. During one of your sessions, your student confides in you that, at a party the previous weekend, they tried a joint. They say this is the first time they have tried it and you believe them. They go on to say that it made them feel good. They felt relaxed, and also worried less about their dad's situation. They are telling you because they feel guilty for using cannabis when their parents have told them not to. How would you respond to them?

Scenario 2: Medical use

You are a family therapist and one of your clients is a family with two kids (M10 and F14). The mother is battling cancer and undergoing chemotherapy, which is why the family was referred to you. During one of your sessions with the family, the mom reveals that she is starting to use cannabis as a part of her treatment to address the side effects of chemotherapy. After her chemo treatment, she smokes a joint on the porch of their home. She also keeps cannabis pre-rolls in the house, as well as cannabis gummies, which she takes at night to help her sleep. Their daughter has been caught using cannabis in the past, at ages 12 and 13. Both times she was out with friends and was caught by local police. She says she has not used cannabis since the second time she was caught at age 13. But, she has also been having a hard time dealing with her mother's illness and the parents are concerned about having cannabis in the home. They are keeping it locked up, but a few times when the daughter has witnessed the mother smoking, she has made comments about how it isn't fair that her mom gets to use it and she gets in trouble for it. The parents want to know how to address this with their daughter. What would you tell them?

Scenario 3: Home from college

You are a substance abuse counselor and receive a call from a very worried dad about his son (M19). While in high school, the son was studious and always made good grades. But he was also a bit of an outsider and had trouble making friends. His dad explains that he is shy, and can be awkward around other people. Last August, his son left for college in another state. During the first semester, he would call and text his parents excited about the new friends he had made and the social acceptance he was experiencing. He often told them about going to parties and football games with his new friends, including a young lady that he likes a lot. After the first semester, the school sent his parents a copy of his report card, and it was not great. Their son, who had earned all As and Bs in high school, was pulling mostly Cs and one D. When they confronted him about it, he got defensive and said he was just adjusting to college life and enjoying his new friends. He promised to do better next semester. Since he had always been a good student, his parents backed off. Then, he came home for the summer in May. A week after he returned, his report card arrived and it was somewhat better than the previous one. He had one C but also Bs and a few As. When he returned home from school, his parents noticed that he smelled like cannabis quite often when he came home after going out, and they also thought he was smoking in his room. They said his eyes were always red, and he seemed to have the "munchies". They live in a state where cannabis is legal, but neither of them have ever used it or brought it into the home. They are worried that his cannabis use, along with a new peer group, may be contributing to his poor grades and that he may flunk out if they don't do something. His mom wants to make him go to inpatient treatment, but his dad is not sure that is the right approach. What would you recommend?

Exercise 3: Understanding the Spectrum of Adolescent Substance Use

This exercise encourages critical thinking, counseling skill development, and harm reduction literacy, preparing students for real-world engagement with adolescents navigating substance use.

Objective

This exercise will help students demonstrate their understanding of the continuum of adolescent substance use and apply harm reduction principles in counseling scenarios.

Instructions

Case Study Analysis (Small Group Activity – 30 Minutes)
   Students will be divided into small groups and given a case study describing a teen's substance use behavior. Each case will align with one of the categories on the continuum: Experimental, Sporadic/Occasional, Regular, Problematic, or Hazardous/Chaotic Use.
   Each group will:

a) Identify where on the continuum the teen's substance use falls.
b) Describe the potential risks and consequences associated with their level of use.
c) Propose harm reduction strategies that could be used to support the teen.

Case Studies

1. Experimental Use – "Mia's First Experience"
   Mia, 15, is at a sleepover with friends when they suggest trying cannabis. She has never used it before but is curious and wants to fit in. She takes a couple of hits from a vape pen

but doesn't enjoy the sensation and decides not to try it again. The next day, she feels fine and doesn't think much about it.
Discussion questions:

- Where does Mia's use fall on the continuum?
- What are the potential risks, even though she only used once?
- How could a harm reduction approach be used to ensure safer decision-making in the future?

2. Sporadic/Occasional Use – "Jordan's Social Drinking"
Jordan, 17, drinks alcohol only at big events like birthdays, prom, or New Year's parties. They never drink alone or on school nights but occasionally drink too much and get sick. Last month, Jordan drank at a party, felt dizzy, and had trouble remembering parts of the night. They are not worried about their drinking because it happens infrequently.
Discussion questions:

- How does Jordan's use fit into the continuum?
- What are the risks of occasional binge drinking?
- How could a counselor introduce harm reduction strategies for safer alcohol use?

3. Regular Use – "Leo's Stress Relief Routine"
Leo, 16, has been smoking cannabis a few times a week after school to relax. At first, it was just with friends, but now he also uses alone to help with stress from school. His grades have dropped slightly, but he doesn't think cannabis is a problem because it helps him unwind. He notices that when he doesn't smoke, he feels more irritable and restless.
Discussion questions:

- Where does Leo's use fall on the continuum?
- What are the potential risks of regular cannabis use, especially for a developing brain?
- How could harm reduction be used to help Leo reflect on his use without pushing abstinence?

4. Problematic Use – "Emily's Daily Vaping"
Emily, 16, started vaping nicotine occasionally but now does it multiple times a day, even during class. She feels anxious and irritable when she doesn't vape and finds herself sneaking away to use it. She has tried to cut back but struggles with cravings. Her parents recently caught her and grounded her, but she continues to vape when she can.
Discussion questions:

- How does Emily's use differ from experimental or occasional use?
- What withdrawal symptoms or dependency signs is she experiencing?
- How could a harm reduction approach support Emily in managing her use?

5. Hazardous/Chaotic Use – "Ricky's Escalating Drug Use"
Ricky, 17, started using prescription opioids recreationally with friends but now takes them almost daily. He has built a tolerance and needs higher doses to feel the same effects. He has experienced withdrawal symptoms, including nausea and body aches, when he doesn't take the pills. Ricky has started skipping school and borrowing money to buy more pills, sometimes lying about why he needs the money.

Discussion questions:

- What signs suggest Ricky's substance use has become hazardous/chaotic?
- What are the short-term and long-term risks associated with opioid use?
- How could a harm reduction strategy help Ricky reduce immediate risks while working toward support?

Role-Playing Counseling Scenarios (Partner Activity – 20 Minutes)

Students will pair up and take turns acting as a counselor and a teen based on the provided case studies. The goal is to practice:

- Nonjudgmental communication
- Harm reduction strategies
- Engagement and goal-setting rather than an abstinence-only approach

For example, one student will play Ricky (from the Hazardous/Chaotic case), and the other will act as the counselor. The counselor might explore safer use options, overdose prevention, or pathways to support Ricky without forcing immediate abstinence.

Reflection and Discussion (20 Minutes)

As a class, discuss:

a) What challenges did you face when identifying substance use patterns?
b) How did harm reduction strategies differ from abstinence-only approaches?
c) How can understanding the continuum help shift counseling practices toward engagement over punishment?

Assessment

Students will submit a one- to two-page reflection on their key takeaways, including:

- How the continuum of use helped them understand adolescent substance use.
- How they would apply harm reduction principles in real-world counseling.
- Any challenges they encountered in thinking about substance use beyond a strict abstinence framework.

Exercise 4: "Walking the Line" – Applying the Safer Use Continuum with Adolescents

Objective

Students will apply the Safer Use Continuum framework (Safe → Safer → Moderate → Controlled Use) to clinical vignettes and practice delivering harm reduction-informed responses tailored to teens and their families.

Part 1: Group Work – Continuum Sorting and Analysis (30 minutes)

In Part 1, you will work in small groups to analyze real-world teen vignettes, identify where each individual falls on the Safer Use Continuum, and explore harm reduction strategies that match their developmental needs and level of risk.

Vignette 1 – "Eddie, 15": Eddie is a sophomore who has never used substances. He's active in theater, has a strong friend group, and is close to his parents. Recently, he told a counselor that he's feeling pressure at parties to try vaping and cannabis. He said, "I don't really want to, but I also don't want to be the only one not doing it." He's asked for advice on "how to say no without looking lame."

- **Prompt for students**:
  Where does Eddie fall on the continuum? What harm reduction strategies could help him maintain his choice while navigating peer pressure?

Vignette 2 – "Mara, 16": Mara has been experimenting with cannabis about once every other week. She mostly uses at home alone to cope with anxiety and sleep issues. She's cautious about where she gets it and always uses clean paraphernalia. She recently read online that vaping THC is "safer" than smoking it. She says she's not addicted, "I just like feeling calm."

- **Prompt for students**:
  Where would you place Mara on the continuum? What safer use strategies are already in place? What are the developmental risks? How would you keep the door open for future conversations?

Vignette 3 – "David, 17": David drinks alcohol most weekends with friends. He says he limits himself to two to three drinks, never drinks on school nights, and always has a designated driver. His parents suspect something but haven't confronted him. David says, "I've got it under control – it's not like I'm getting blackout drunk or doing it every day."

- **Prompt for students**:
  How would you determine whether David is practicing controlled use or simply rationalizing risk? What language would you use to engage him in a harm reduction conversation? How might developmental factors complicate "control"?

Vignette 4 – "Erica, 14": Erica recently had a serious scare after mixing her brother's Adderall with alcohol at a party. She vomited and passed out but didn't tell her parents. Since then, she's avoided parties but still experiments occasionally with substances her friends bring to school. She doesn't understand why mixing was dangerous and jokes that she "can handle it better now."

- **Prompt for students**:
  Where does Erica fall on the continuum? What harm reduction education is needed here? How would you address risk without triggering shame or defensiveness?

Vignette 5 – "Jack, 16": Jack smokes cannabis daily, usually before and after school. He says it helps with his ADHD symptoms, which he feels aren't being addressed by his current treatment plan. He's been caught twice by school staff and is on probation. He says, "I don't want to stop – I just want people to stop freaking out."

- **Prompt for students**:
  Where does Jack fall on the continuum? What are the limitations of moderate or controlled use in this case? How can harm reduction principles be applied in a context that also includes legal or school consequences?

Student Instructions:

- In small groups (3–4), read each vignette.
- Place each teen on the Safer Use Continuum (Safe, Safer, Moderate, Controlled).
- Justify the placement: Which clues support your categorization? What individual/contextual factors (e.g., mental health, family dynamics, impulsivity) influenced your decision?
- Identify one harm reduction strategy appropriate to the teen's position on the continuum.
- Note developmental concerns or caveats for working with adolescents at this point on the continuum.
- **Deliverable**: Groups briefly present one case and their rationale to the class (1–2 minutes each).

Part 2: Role-Play – Counseling a Teen or Parent (20 minutes)

1. **Set-Up**:
   - Students pair up. One plays a counselor, the other a teen or concerned parent.
   - Each pair selects or is assigned one of the vignettes from Part 1.

2. **Instructions**:
   - The "counselor" practices engaging the client using harm reduction principles:
     - Meet them where they are.
     - Use nonjudgmental, motivational language.
     - Avoid abstinence-only framing unless clinically appropriate.
     - Acknowledge the client's concerns and goals.
     - Explore safer use strategies or small steps toward change.
     - The "client" improvises based on the vignette and responds authentically.

3. **Debrief in Pairs**:
   - What was challenging?
   - What language felt affirming or dismissive?
   - How did you incorporate the continuum concept without labeling or pressuring?

Part 3: Wrap-Up Discussion (10 minutes)

Whole-class reflection:

- How did applying the continuum change your approach compared to an abstinence-based mindset?
- What are some ways to integrate this framework when working with caregivers who may be more rigid?
- What challenges might arise when assessing where a teen falls on the continuum?

Exercise 5: Practicing Motivational Interviewing with a Mandated Client

In this exercise, you will have the opportunity to apply MI skills in a realistic scenario. You'll be working with the case of Noah, a 16-year-old who was suspended for selling cannabis at school and is now mandated to treatment. Noah isn't seeking help voluntarily and comes into the conversation defensive and skeptical.

Of course, your goal isn't to "fix" Noah or convince him to stop using cannabis. Instead, you will practice using MI to build rapport, explore ambivalence, and support his autonomy. You will rotate roles – therapist, client, and observer – and work together to notice what helps reduce resistance, elicit change talk, and foster engagement without pushing an agenda.

This exercise is about learning to meet teens where they are, using a respectful, collaborative stance – even when motivation is externally imposed. Expect some discomfort, some creativity, and a chance to try out language and strategies in a supportive environment.

Scenario: Noah, a 16-Year-Old Caught Selling Cannabis at School

Objective: Students will practice applying Motivational Interviewing (MI) strategies with an adolescent client who is mandated to treatment and initially resistant. The focus is on building rapport, exploring ambivalence, eliciting change talk, and collaboratively identifying harm reduction strategies within a developmentally appropriate framework.

Step 1: Case Overview (10 minutes)

Background:

Noah is a 16-year-old high school junior who was caught selling cannabis to peers on school grounds. He was suspended and is now mandated to attend a substance use evaluation before being considered for reentry. Noah downplays the incident, saying selling weed is "not a big deal", that "everyone smokes", and that he was just trying to make some money. He's irritated about being forced into treatment and distrustful of adults. At the same time, he admits that his mom is "really pissed", and he's worried about being labeled a criminal or getting kicked out of school permanently.

Small Group Discussion Prompts:

- What stage of change is Noah likely in?
- What developmental and contextual factors might be influencing his behavior?
- What counselor judgments might arise?
- What specific MI strategies can you use to engage a teen who is externally motivated without increasing resistance or shutting down the conversation?

Step 2: Role Play (25 minutes total)

Format: Groups of 3–4. Rotate roles:

- Therapist
- Client (Noah)
- Observer(s)

Client (Noah) Prompt Sheet:

- You're here because you have to be.
- You don't think it was a big deal – you weren't hurting anyone.
- You're annoyed about being suspended.
- You think adults overreact and don't get it.
- You don't plan to stop smoking or selling, but you don't want to get in trouble again.

Therapist Goals:

Use MI to:

- Acknowledge resistance and build rapport.
- Explore ambivalence about cannabis and the consequences of the incident.
- Develop discrepancy between current behavior and future goals or personal values.
- Identify harm reduction strategies (e.g., not selling at school, avoiding risky situations).
- Reinforce autonomy and self-efficacy.

Observer Feedback Checklist:

- Did the therapist express empathy without judgment?
- Did they use reflective listening and affirmations?
- Did they avoid the righting reflex?
- Did they elicit any change talk?
- Did they reinforce client autonomy?

Step 3: Group Debrief (15–20 minutes)

Whole-Class Discussion Prompts:

- What MI strategies helped reduce Noah's resistance?
- What approaches were effective in building trust?
- What specific language or tone encouraged engagement?
- How did you balance acknowledging legal/school consequences without being punitive?
- How could harm reduction be framed in a way that feels realistic and relevant to Noah?

Optional Written Reflection Prompt:

In 1–2 paragraphs, reflect on:

- What felt most effective in working with Noah?
- What was challenging about staying in the MI stance?
- How would you adjust your approach if you had a second session with him?

Summary

This classroom exercise illustrates how MI can be applied in a real-world context with a resistant adolescent who is mandated to treatment. Noah, a 16-year-old suspended for selling cannabis at school, enters the session frustrated, distrustful, and lacking internal motivation for change. Rather than confronting his behavior, students practice using MI to build rapport, validate his perspective, and elicit his own motivations for avoiding future consequences. Through open-ended questions, reflective listening, and a harm reduction lens, students explore how MI supports adolescent autonomy while promoting insight and behavior change. The exercise highlights the importance of meeting teens where they are and working collaboratively – even when the client is not seeking help voluntarily.

Exercise 6: Parent-Teen Communication Using CRAFT and MI Skills

Objective

By practicing these communication techniques, students gain a deeper understanding of how to help parents shift from reactive, fear-based responses to more effective, relationship-building conversations. This reinforces autonomy, trust, and incremental change rather than confrontation and control

Activity 1: Practicing Reflective Listening

Overview:
When parents discover their teen is engaging in risky behavior, such as substance use, their instinct may be to lecture, criticize, or problem-solve immediately. However, these reactions often shut down conversation rather than opening space for meaningful dialogue. Reflective listening helps parents stay engaged without judgment, allowing their teen to feel heard and reducing defensiveness. This technique involves summarizing or paraphrasing what the teen says in a way that conveys understanding and encourages further discussion.

Parent-Teen Role-Play Scenarios:

- Scenario 1: A 16-year-old, Jordan, says: *"I only smoke weed because it helps with my stress. You don't get it."*
- Scenario 2: A 17-year-old, Maya, says: *"I don't need you to tell me how to live my life. You always assume the worst about me."*
- Scenario 3: A 15-year-old, Sam, says: *"It's not a big deal. All my friends drink. It's just normal."*

Student Activity:

- One student plays the parent, the other plays the teen.
- The "parent" must respond with reflective listening rather than arguing or lecturing.
- After each round, switch roles and discuss:
  - What responses felt effective?
  - How did reflective listening change the conversation?

Activity 2: Using "Change Talk" to Guide Conversations

Overview:
Rather than telling a teen what they "should" do, parents can encourage "change talk" – statements from the teen that show openness to change. Motivational Interviewing techniques, such as asking open-ended questions and affirming positive behaviors, help guide the teen toward their own reasons for making healthier choices.

Parent-Teen Role-Play Scenarios:

- Scenario 1: Chris, 18, says: *"I don't think drinking is that bad – it's just how people have fun."*
- Scenario 2: Tessa, 17, says: *"I can quit anytime I want. It's not like I'm addicted or anything."*
- Scenario 3: Eric, 16, says: *"You and Dad are always on my case. It just makes me want to do it more."*

Student Activity:

- One student plays the parent, the other plays the teen.
- The "parent" must use open-ended questions to encourage the teen to express any concerns or ambivalence they have about their substance use.
- After role-play, discuss:
  - Did the "parent" successfully elicit change talk?
  - What strategies helped the teen reflect on their choices?

Activity 3: Reinforcing Positive Behaviors

Overview:
When a teen is struggling with substance use, parents often focus only on negative behaviors. However, reinforcing small, positive changes can be more effective in guiding behavior than punishment. Parents can learn to notice and acknowledge behaviors that align with their teen's values and long-term goals, helping to increase motivation for healthier choices.

Parent-Teen Role-Play Scenarios:

- Scenario 1: Alex, 17, has been skipping school regularly but attends all his classes today.
- Scenario 2: Jamie, 16, typically stays out late but comes home on time for the first time in weeks.
- Scenario 3: Ryan, 18, has been using cannabis daily but mentions going two days without it.

Student Activity:

- One student plays the parent, the other plays the teen.
- The "parent" must use positive reinforcement without sounding patronizing.
- After role-play, discuss:
  - How did the "teen" react to reinforcement?
  - What approaches felt most effective?

Activity 4: De-escalating Conflict

Overview:
Many conversations between parents and teens become power struggles, especially when substance use or risky behavior is involved. Parents often escalate the situation by reacting emotionally, leading to shutdown or rebellion from the teen. Learning to de-escalate conflict by staying calm, setting boundaries, and choosing when to engage in discussion is a critical skill.

Parent-Teen Role-Play Scenarios:

- Scenario 1: Sophia, 16, storms into the house and yells: *"You're so controlling! You don't get to tell me what to do!"*
- Scenario 2: Malik, 17, comes home high. When confronted, he says: *"It's my life – I'll do what I want!"*
- Scenario 3: Eva, 15, breaks curfew and, when asked about it, responds sarcastically: *"Oh, I didn't realize I had a bedtime like a little kid."*

Student Activity:

- One student plays the parent, the other plays the teen.
- The "parent" must practice staying calm and de-escalating instead of reacting emotionally.
- After role-play, discuss:
  - What responses prevented the situation from escalating?
  - How did de-escalation affect the "teen's" willingness to engage?

Activity 5: Avoiding Conversational Traps

Overview:
Teens sometimes use manipulation, guilt trips, or blame to avoid accountability. Parents may fall into the trap of arguing, defending, or over-explaining rather than setting firm but supportive boundaries. Learning to stay neutral and set limits without escalating is an essential skill for parents.

Parent-Teen Role-Play Scenarios:

- Scenario 1: Mateo, 18, asks for money and, when refused, says: *"You don't trust me! You always treat me like a little kid."*
- Scenario 2: Zoe, 17, wants to go to an unsupervised party and says: *"If you really loved me, you'd let me go."*
- Scenario 3: Dylan, 16, gets caught drinking and blames the parent: *"Well, maybe if you weren't so strict, I wouldn't feel like I have to hide things from you!"*

Student Activity:

- One student plays the parent, the other plays the teen.
- The "parent" must avoid arguing, defending, or giving in to guilt trips while still maintaining a connection.
- After role-play, discuss:
  - What responses allowed the parent to hold a boundary without escalating the conflict?
  - How did the teen respond when the parent refused to engage in a power struggle?

Final Reflection Questions for Students

- What patterns did you notice in how you instinctively responded in the "parent" role?
- Which skills felt natural, and which were more difficult?
- How do these techniques align with harm reduction and motivational interviewing approaches?
- How can you support parents in using these strategies effectively in real-world situations?

Conclusion and Key Takeaways

Conclusion

As a philosophy, harm reduction was born out of the belief that everyone, even people who use drugs (PWUD), should have access to programs that help them lead safer lives. While harm reduction approaches such as bike helmets and seatbelts are largely accepted and supported, programs and policies related to substance use have faced continual backlash. The belief that the only goal related to substance use should be abstinence and that all illicit substance use constitutes abuse has stood in the way of rational, evidence-informed policies on the use of drugs. The continued criminalization of PWUD and the claim that anything not rooted in abstinence is encouraging drug use has made the adoption of harm reduction based policies and programs extremely difficult, especially in the United States. Even so, many scholars and clinicians recognize the value in taking a harm reduction approach as it is rooted in humanity, pragmatism and reflective of the research on substance use and change.

One key to understand harm reduction is the reality of substance use as a continuum of behavior. Rather than an "all use is abuse" approach, harm reduction recognizes that there are many patterns of substance use, from experimentation to chaotic use. For the therapist, this means that it is important to determine where their client is on this spectrum, as well as what the risks associated with each type of use are. Only then can risk reduction commence and work can be done to ensure safer use. However, as discussed, accepting substance use, especially illicit substance use, as a continuum is especially difficult when working with adolescent clients.

Adolescent substance use is particularly tricky when it comes to harm reduction. The paternalistic nature of adolescent based interventions, combined with the Just Say No focused messaging, encourages interventions to be nothing but abstinence focused where the substance use is the star of the show. In reality, problematic substance use among the adolescent population is often an attempt to treat physical, psychological, or social sources of pain or trauma. The cornerstone of a harm reduction focused approach when working with adolescents is getting a holistic view of their lives and sources of risk and resilience. Another key component is involving the adolescent in the decisions regarding their goals for treatment, even if those goals do not include abstinence. As the harm reduction paradigm reveals, there are ways to improve and make the lives of people who use substances safer, even if they are actively using. And while abstinence may be the smartest choice for adolescents, it is not always the one that they make. By starting where the client is, therapists can monitor their safety and decisions while encouraging behaviors that will reduce risk, while also helping them address the source of their pain.

Key takeaways

1. *Harm reduction exists because of a desire to improve the lives and safety of those who engage in risky behavior.* From sex, to driving, to riding a bike, we all participate in behaviors that pose risks. For most risky behaviors, we do not demand abstention because of risk, but rather create tools (e.g., condoms, bike helmets, seat belts) that reduce the risk of engaging in the behavior. However, with drugs, the moral beliefs about substance use result in the demanding of abstinence as the only way to address risk. The history of harm reduction follows the community's desire to reduce the risks of sexual activity and substance use with the goal of reducing the transmission of HIV.
2. *Harm reduction programs like syringe access, overdose prevention facilities, drug user's unions and drug checking services aim to reduce the risks of using substances and empower people who use drugs to actively participate in policy making and education.* The potential harms addressed by these programs include infection and the transmission of blood-borne diseases, fatal overdose, and the ingestion of contaminated substances. Research supports the success of these programs in reducing risk, however, the beliefs about the morality of substance use and the inability of harm reduction to stop it, has resulted in historic pushback to harm reduction-based programs, especially in the United States. These programs have been almost impossible to implement and fund due to beliefs about people who use drugs and how such programs enable drug use.
3. *While drug use among adolescents exists, outside of alcohol and cannabis, it is very rare, as is the admission into drug treatment.* The ways in which alcohol is treated in national use surveys compared to illicit substances illustrates the belief that "all use is abuse" when it comes to illicit substances but not alcohol, even though all are illegal for those under 21. Drug using patterns have traditionally ebbed and flowed over time, however, in recent years, they have been in decline. Notable is that the rates of cannabis use have not increased, even after legalization began to occur. Also, use rates remained stable even as perceived risk decreased and perceived availability increased.
4. *There are very real risks and potential harms for adolescents who use substances.* Adolescence is a vulnerable period due to brain development, psychological experiences and the social environment. These areas of an adolescent's life can play off each other and raise the risks associated with using psychoactive substances. This risk increases the younger the initiation into substance use. Impulsivity, lack of critical and long-term thinking, the gradual development of emotional intelligence, and psychological resilience along with peer influences can influence the impact of substance use. There are programs that take a holistic and nonjudgmental approach that have found success in improving the lives of adolescents who use substances by addressing the factors unique to this time of life.
5. *The War on Drugs narratives have shaped a treatment landscape dominated by criminalization, abstinence-only models, and coercive interventions – often reinforcing stigma, limiting access to care, and undermining adolescent development.* This paradigm, which includes the criminalization of substance use, the introduction of the disease model of treatment and concepts like "tough love" is in direct conflict with harm reduction, which prioritizes safety, autonomy, and relational support. These prohibition-based approaches have influenced families, schools, and communities, and often perpetuate punitive practices such as zero-tolerance discipline and court-mandated treatment.
6. *The key principles of harm reduction as a therapeutic intervention include meeting clients where they are, building strong therapeutic alliances, and recognizing substance use as a*

relationship rather than a moral failing. This approach helps de-stigmatize use, increase engagement, and address the psychosocial factors driving behavior. Emphasis is placed on the Stages of Change (SOC) model and the need to reduce fear and increase hope for families navigating adolescent substance use within a harm reduction framework.

7. *Practicing Harm Reduction Therapy (HRT) involves more than adopting new techniques; it requires a shift in how clinicians conceptualize change, ethics, and the therapeutic relationship*. Principles such as infinite flexibility, radical neutrality, and the dialectical stance are needed when working with clients at various stages of readiness. Moving beyond abstinence-based models allows for more ethical, person-centered care, particularly when clients are not ready or able to pursue abstinence. There is a need for ongoing self-awareness among therapists so that they may advocate for more flexible, client-centered approaches to evaluating treatment effectiveness. HRT is both a clinical practice and a worldview grounded in respect, collaboration, and doing no harm.

8. *Moving beyond abstinence-based approaches, HRT challenges therapists to adopt principles such as infinite flexibility, radical neutrality, and cultural responsiveness while navigating risk, autonomy, and engagement*. Core tensions in HRT exist, such as structure versus process, initiating versus responding, and behavioral focus versus emotional depth. Therapist self-awareness, ethical decision-making, and client-centered collaboration are key. As is the ongoing need to adapt HRT to diverse cultural contexts. By meeting adolescents where they are, HRT fosters trust, reduces harm, and supports meaningful engagement without coercion.

9. *Integrating harm reduction principles with developmental science and parenting theory can equip families to more effectively support adolescents navigating substance use and mental health challenges*. Authoritative parenting, which balances warmth and structure, is emphasized as a protective factor that aligns with teens' needs for autonomy, identity formation, and emotional regulation is an important aspect of healthy development. Harm reduction is not only a clinical model but a parenting approach that fosters open communication, mutual respect, and realistic goal setting.

10. *Harm reduction therapy (HRT) aligns with adolescent development and parenting, offering an alternative to traditional abstinence-based approaches*. Teens' risk-taking and identity formation are natural, not pathological. Harm reduction meets youth where they are, reducing stigma and fostering engagement through nonjudgmental, client-centered care. By empowering teens and families to set collaborative, realistic goals, HRT builds trust and fosters long-term behavioral change. Also of importance are family systems, cultural context, and the need for developmentally appropriate, trauma-informed responses.

11. *The Integrated Dynamic Engagement Assessment (IDEA) offers a developmentally responsive, client-centered alternative to traditional diagnostic assessment models in adolescent substance use treatment*. Rather than assuming a linear path toward abstinence, IDEA frames assessment as an ongoing, collaborative process that unfolds across multiple life domains. It emphasizes engagement, safety, and curiosity, helping clinicians understand the "why" of substance use in relation to identity, neurodevelopment, trauma, and social context. This approach allows for flexible intervention strategies, whether teens are experimenting, using regularly, or navigating chaotic use patterns.

12. *There is a deep interconnection between trauma and adolescent substance use, framing substance use not as defiance or pathology, but as an adaptive response to emotional overwhelm, relational wounds, and systemic harm*. Trauma-informed approaches integrate compassion, flexibility, and developmental attunement into substance use treatment.

These models center emotional safety, collaboration, and respect for the protective functions of substance use, even when abstinence is not the goal. Clinical adaptations for adolescents emphasize creative engagement, emotion regulation skills, and attention to social context and attachment. Grounded in attachment theory, this approach offers a developmentally appropriate, client-centered pathway for healing that honors the complexity of adolescent lives.

13. *The integration of CRAFT (Community Reinforcement and Family Training) with harm reduction provides a relational, developmentally attuned framework for fostering safety, engagement, and sustainable progress.* CRAFT is a harm reduction–oriented approach for engaging parents of adolescents and young adults with substance use and co-occurring mental health challenges. It provides empirically supported strategies to improve communication, reinforce non–substance-using behavior, and promote family resilience, without confrontation or ultimatums. In addition to empowering caregivers, CRAFT-informed approaches can significantly expand therapists' clinical toolkits, offering structured, flexible methods for supporting families across a wide range of developmental and diagnostic presentations.

Final thoughts

In a time when the fear about a teen using substances immediately conjures up images of a life without success and potential squandered, it is important that the therapist takes in the whole view. Adolescence is a time of great change, vulnerability, and opportunity. And while substance use at any age presents a level of risk, the heightened level of risk that exists during adolescence should not cloud the desire to see the full picture. Starting where the client is, focusing on safety and listening to how the client would like to make change and what they need to feel safe and secure should outshine the reaction to substance use. Understanding where a teen is on the continuum of use, immediate threats to their health and safety, and how use fits into the context of their physical, psychological, and social lives is harm reduction. It is common sense, public health, and the way to help teens make lasting, positive change.

Appendix A

Eight general harm reduction principles from Harm Reduction Coalition

https://harmreduction.org/about-us/principles-of-harm-reduction/

1. Accepts, for better or worse, that licit and illicit drug use is part of our world and chooses to work to minimize its harmful effects rather than simply ignore or condemn them.
2. Understands drug use as a complex, multi-faceted phenomenon that encompasses a continuum of behaviors from severe use to total abstinence, and acknowledges that some ways of using drugs are clearly safer than others.
3. Establishes quality of individual and community life and well-being – not necessarily cessation of all drug use – as the criteria for successful interventions and policies.
4. Calls for the non-judgmental, non-coercive provision of services and resources to people who use drugs and the communities in which they live in order to assist them in reducing attendant harm.
5. Ensures that people who use drugs and those with a history of drug use routinely have a real voice in the creation of programs and policies designed to serve them.
6. Affirms people who use drugs (PWUD) themselves as the primary agents of reducing the harms of their drug use and seeks to empower PWUD to share information and support each other in strategies which meet their actual conditions of use.
7. Recognizes that the realities of poverty, class, racism, social isolation, past trauma, sex-based discrimination, and other social inequalities affect both people's vulnerability to and capacity for effectively dealing with drug-related harm.
8. Does not attempt to minimize or ignore the real and tragic harm and danger that can be associated with illicit drug use.

Appendix B

Resources

Community Reinforcement and Family Training (CRAFT)

The CRAFT Treatment Manual for Substance Use Problems: Working with Family Members:
This manual provides a comprehensive guide to implementing the CRAFT program. Designed for clinicians, it offers structured yet flexible strategies to assist concerned significant others (CSOs) in encouraging treatment entry for individuals resistant to seeking help for substance use problems. The manual includes step-by-step implementation guidelines, case examples, sample dialogues, troubleshooting tips, and 28 reproducible forms and handouts, equipping practitioners with practical tools to support both clients and their families.

Smith, J. E., & Meyers, R. J. (2023). *The CRAFT Treatment Manual for Substance Use Problems: Working with family members*. Guilford Press.

CRAFT Trainings:
Developer of CRAFT Dr. Robert J. Meyers offers several pathways for professionals seeking certification:

Clinician Certification: This process involves comprehensive training, including access to an online curriculum with step-by-step guides for conducting CRAFT sessions with fidelity. Clinicians receive client worksheets and session preparation modules to support their practice. Upon successful completion, participants are awarded a certificate as a certified CRAFT clinician.

- Supervisor Certification: For certified clinicians aiming to train and certify others within their agencies, the supervisor certification provides additional training focused on sustaining high-fidelity CRAFT services. This certification enables supervisors to ensure the quality and consistency of CRAFT implementation within their organizations.
- Intensive Training Services: Dr. Meyers and his associates offer intensive, customized training services designed to meet the specific needs of agencies. The goal is to help participants feel comfortable and confident with the CRAFT model, enabling immediate application with clients.

  Meyers, R. J. (n.d.). *Robert J. Meyers, Ph.D. – Community reinforcement training*. https://www.robertjmeyersphd.com/craft-cra-acra-professional-training

- Online Training Programs: In collaboration with We The Village, Dr. Meyers offers online CRAFT training programs tailored for both professionals and families. These programs combine automated online lessons with virtual live sessions, providing flexible and accessible training options. They are clinically validated and have been proven to help families recover and professionals achieve effective client outcomes.

Meyers, R. J. (n.d.). *Self-guided online CRAFT Training Program*. We The Village. https://www.robertjmeyersphd.com/training/self-guided-online-craft-training-program

Books:

Denning, P., & Little, J. (2012). *Practicing harm reduction psychotherapy: An alternative approach to addictions* (2nd ed.). Guilford Press.

A comprehensive text that serves as a de facto "bible" for practitioners, it is a foundational resource for our book's exploration of harm reduction principles and their application to a model of HRT

Denning, P., & Little, J. (2012). *Over the influence: The harm reduction guide to controlling your drug and alcohol use* (2nd ed.). Guilford Press.

A user-friendly resource for both professionals and lay people, offering practical, nonjudgmental strategies for understanding and managing substance use through a harm reduction lens.

Tatarsky, A. (2002) *Harm reduction psychotherapy: A new treatment for drug and alcohol problems*. Jason Aronson, Inc.

As one of the early architects of harm reduction therapy, Tatarsky structures the book around detailed case examples, offering both clinical depth and practical application – making it highly relevant for readers of our book who are interested in understanding how HRT works in diverse case scenarios.

Foote, J., Wilkens, C., Kosanke, N., & Higgs, S. (2014). *Beyond addiction: How science and kindness help people change*. Scribner, New York.

Grounded in CRAFT principles, *Beyond Addiction* can serve as a reference source for many of the ideas and concepts discussed in this book.

Foote, J., Carpenter, K., & Wilkens, Ca. (2022). *The Beyond Addiction Workbook for Family and Friends: Evidence-based skills to help a loved one make positive change*. New Harbinger.

The Beyond Addiction Workbook for Family and Friends is a companion to *Beyond Addiction* that offers a structured, skill-based guide for families and friends seeking to support a loved one through substance use and related challenges. Based on the Invitation to Change Approach, the workbook integrates principles from CRAFT, Motivational Interviewing, and Acceptance and Commitment Therapy (ACT). It provides exercises, reflection prompts, and communication strategies designed to reduce conflict, build connection, and support behavior change.

Family Support and Peer Services:

SMART Recovery Family & Friends

This mutual aid program offers support for those affected by a loved one's addictive behaviors. Grounded in principles of CBT and CRAFT, it provides practical tools to improve communication, set healthy boundaries, and foster change. With a robust network of both online and in-person meetings, SMART Recovery ensures accessibility and flexibility for participants seeking support. https://smartrecovery.org/family

SMART Recovery Family & Friends Handbook
This structured, user-friendly companion to the SMART Recovery Family & Friends program integrates tools from SMART Recovery and core elements of the CRAFT model, including modules on positive communication, healthy boundaries, problem-solving, and strategies for self-care and emotional regulation. The handbook includes exercises, worksheets, and reflection prompts tailored for use alongside SMART Recovery's mutual aid meetings, both online and in person. https://shop.smartrecovery.org/products/smart-family-friends-handbook

Partnership to End Addiction
A national nonprofit offering CRAFT-informed, peer-led support services for families impacted by substance use, including trained parent coaches, a helpline, and online support groups. Their approach embraces the power of lived experience in fostering change. https://drugfree.org

Harm Reduction Works (HRW)
HRW was developed by HRH413, a grassroots organization advancing harm reduction services and leadership development, and offers a peer-led, harm reduction-based mutual aid model with scripted, exercise-driven meetings – including ones specifically for family and loved ones – that emphasize compassion, connection, and shared learning, and create inclusive spaces for support, education, and community building around substance use and related challenges. https://www.hrh413.org/foundationsstart-here-2

Bibliography

Abraham, A. J., Andrews, C. M., Yingling, M. E., & Shannon, J. (2020). Geographic disparities in availability of opioid use disorder treatment for Medicaid enrollees. *Health Services Research*, *55*(1), 42–51. https://doi.org/10.1111/1475-6773.13242

Ainsworth, M. D. S., Blehar, M. C., Waters, E., & Wall, S. (1978). *Patterns of attachment: A psychological study of the strange situation*. Erlbaum.

Alcoholics Anonymous. (2001). *Alcoholics Anonymous: The story of how many thousands of men and women have recovered from alcoholism* (4th ed.). Alcoholics Anonymous World Services.

Alcoholics Anonymous. (2025). https://www.aa.org/what-is-aa

Alexander, B. K. (2008). *The globalization of addiction: A study in poverty of the spirit*. Oxford University Press. (This book expands on the ideas from the Rat Park study, exploring addiction as a global issue influenced by social and economic factors.)

Amazon.com (2025). *Rapid Response Fentanyl Test Strips*. https://www.amazon.com/BTNX-Rapid-Response-Fentanyl-Strips/dp/B0B64BZ3FV?th=1

American Civil Liberties Union. (April 16, 2020). *A tale of two countries: Racially targeted arrests in the era of marijuana reform*. https://www.aclu.org/publications/tale-two-countries-racially-targeted-arrests-era-marijuana-reform

American Psychiatric Association. (2022). *Diagnostic and statistical manual of mental disorders* (5th ed., text rev.; DSM-5-TR). American Psychiatric Publishing.

American Psychological Association. (n.d.-a). *Cognitive behavioral therapy (CBT)* [Patient and family information sheet]. https://www.apa.org/ptsd-guideline/patients-and-families/cognitive-behavioral.pdf

American Psychological Association. (n.d.-b). Counseling psychology. American Psychological Association. https://www.apa.org/ed/graduate/specialize/counseling

Anderson, K., & Smith, A. W. (2022). *BETTER IS BETTER!: Stories of alcohol harm reduction*. Independently Published.

Aspinall, E. J., Nambiar, D., Goldberg, D. J., Hickman, M., Weir, A., Van Velzen, E., ... Hutchinson, S. J. (2014). Are needle and syringe programmes associated with a reduction in HIV transmission among people who inject drugs: A systematic review and meta-analysis. *International Journal of Epidemiology*, *43*(1), 235–248. doi: 10.1093/ije/dyt243

Attaiaa, L., Beck, F., Richard, J., Marimoutou, C., & Mayet, A., (2016). Relationships between substance initiation sequence and further substance use: A French nationwide retrospective study. *Addictive Behaviors*, 1–5.

Australian Government. (2024). *Online Safety Amendment (Minors and News Media Codes) Act 2024*. Federal Register of Legislation. https://www.legislation.gov.au/C2024A00127/asmade/text

Barry, C. L., Huskamp, H. A., & Goldman, H. H. (2014). A political history of federal mental health and addiction insurance parity. *Health Affairs*, *33*(10), 1606–1617. https://doi.org/10.1377/hlthaff.2014.0163

Baumrind, D. (1966). Effects of authoritative parental control on child behavior. *Child Development*, *37*(4), 887–907.

Bava, S., & Tapert, S. F. (2010). Adolescent brain development and the risk for alcohol and other drug problems. *Neuropsychology Review*, *20*(4), 398–413. https://doi.org/10.1007/s11065-010-9146-6

Bazazi, A. R. Commentary on Rafful et al. (2018). Unpacking involuntary interventions for people who use drugs. Addiction. June, *113*(6), 1064–1065. doi: 10.1111/add.14202. PMID: 29732697; PMCID: PMC7006027.

Beletsky, L., Baker, P., Arredondo, J., Emuka, A., Goodman-Meza, D., Medina-Mora, M., ... Magis-Rodriguez, C. (2018). The global health and equity imperative for safe consumption facilities. *The Lancet*, *392*(10147), 553–554.

Bigg, D. (2001). Substance use management: A harm reduction-principled approach to assisting the relief of drug-related problems. *Journal of Psychoactive Drugs*, *33*(1), 33–38. doi: 10.1080/02791072.2001.10400466

Bond, L., Butler, H., Thomas, L., Carlin, J., Glover, S., Bowes, G., & Patton, G. (2007). Social and school connectedness in early secondary school as predictors of late teenage substance use, mental health and academic outcomes. *Journal of Adolescent Health*, *40*: 356–366.

Bowen, M. (1978). *Family therapy in clinical practice*. Jason Aronson.

Bowlby, J. (1988). *A secure base: Parent-child attachment and healthy human development*. Basic Books.

Brehm, J. W. (1966). *A theory of psychological reactance*. Academic Press.

Brehm, S. S., & Brehm, J. W. (1981). *Psychological reactance: A theory of freedom and control*. Academic Press.

Bryant, A., Schulenberg, J., O'Malley, P., Bachman, J., & Johnston, L. (2003). How academic achievement, attitudes and behaviors relate to the course of substance use during adolescence: A 6-year, multiwave national longitudinal study. *Journal of Research on Adolescence*, *13*(3), 361–397.

Bureau of Justice Statistics. (2024). National Prisoner Statistics. https://bjs.ojp.gov/data-collection/national-prisoner-statistics-nps

Cadet, J. L., Bisagno, V., & Milroy, C. M. (2018). Editorial: Long-term consequences of adolescent drug use: Evidence from pre-clinical and clinical models. *Frontiers in Behavioral Neuroscience*, 12, Article 83. https://doi.org/10.3389/fnbeh.2018.00083

California Age-Appropriate Design Code Act, Cal. Civ. Code § 1798.99.28 (2022). https://leginfo.legislature.ca.gov/faces/billTextClient.xhtml?bill_id=202120220AB2273

California Health Care Foundation. (2022). *Fragmented care harms people with mental illness and substance use disorder*. https://www.chcf.org/publication/fragmented-care-harms-people-mental-illness-substance-use-disorder/

Carson, E. A., & Kluckow, R. (2023). *Prisoners in 2022-Statistical tables*. Bureau of Justice Statistics.

Catalano, R., Fagan, A., Gavin, L., Greenberg, M., Irwin, C., Ross, D., & Shek, D. (2012). Worldwide application of prevention science in adolescent health. *Lancet*, *379*(9826), 1653–1664.

Catalano, R., Kosterman, R., Hawkins, J., Newcomb, M., & Abbott, R. (1996). Modeling the etiology of adolescent substance use: A test of the social development model. *Journal of Drug Issues*, *26*(2), 429–455.

Center for Public Health Law Research. (2023). *Good Samaritan overdose prevention laws dataset*. Prescription Drug Abuse Policy System. https://pdaps.org/datasets/good-samaritan-overdose-laws-1501695153

Center for Public Justice. (n.d.). *Classroom or courtroom? Problems & solutions to the school-to-prison pipeline*. https://cpjustice.org/classroom-or-courtroom-problems-solutions-to-the-school-to-prison-pipeline/

Centers for Disease Control and Prevention. (2022, August). *Teen newsletter: Concussions*. David J. Sencer CDC Museum. https://www.cdc.gov/museum/education/newsletter/2022/aug/index.html

Centers for Disease Control and Prevention. (2025). *What you can do to test for fentanyl*. https://www.cdc.gov/stop-overdose/safety/index.html

Claborn, K., Samora, J., McCormick, K., Whittfield, Q., Courtois, F., Lozada, K., ... Potter, J. (2023). "We do it ourselves": Strengths and opportunities for improving the practice of harm reduction. *Harm Reduction Journal*, *20*, 70–84.

Cohen, A., Vakharia, S., Netherland, J., & Frederique, K. (2022). How the war on drugs impacts social determinants of health beyond the criminal legal system, *Annals of Medicine*, *54*: 2024–2038.

Collins, S., & Clifaseri, S. (2023). Harm reduction treatment for substance use. *Advances in Psychotherapy-Evidence Based Practice*, Volume 49. Newburyport, MA: Hogrefe Publishing.

Comas-Díaz, L., Hall, G. N., & Neville, H. A. (2019). Racial trauma: Theory, research, and healing: Introduction to the special issue. *American Psychologist, 74*(1), 1–5. https://doi.org/10.1037/amp0000442

Comprehensive Opioid, Stimulant, and Substance Use Program. (n.d.). *Harm reduction.* COSSUP Resource Center. https://www.cossup.org/Topics/HarmReduction/

Craig, S. L., Eaton, A. D., McInroy, L. B., Leung, V. W. Y., & Krishnan, S. (2021). Can affirmative cognitive-behavioral therapy (CBT) improve health outcomes for LGBTQ+ youth? A meta-analysis. *Journal of Youth and Adolescence, 50*(5), 893–907.

Cruz, O. S. (2015). Nonproblematic illegal drug use: Drug use management strategies in a Portuguese sample. *Journal of Drug Issues, 45*(2), 133–150. https://doi.org/10.1177/0022042614559842

DanceSafe. (2025). *Drug checking.* https://dancesafe.org/drug-checking/

Dean, S., Britt, E., Bell, E., Stanley, J., & Collings, S. (2016). Motivational interviewing to enhance adolescent mental health treatment engagement: A randomized clinical trial. *Psychological Medicine, 46*(9), 1961–1969. https://doi.org/10.1017/S0033291716000568

Debenham, J., Champion, K., Birrell, L., & Newton, N. (2022). Effectiveness of a neuroscience-based harm reduction program for older adolescents: A cluster randomised controlled trial of The Illicit Project. *Preventative Medicine Reports, 26*, 1–7.

Denning, P., & Little, J. (2012). *Practicing harm reduction psychotherapy: An alternative approach to addictions* (2nd ed.). Guilford Press.

Denning, P., & Little, J. (2017). *Over the influence: The harm reduction guide to controlling your drug and alcohol use* (2nd ed.). Guilford Press.

Des Jarlais, D.C. (2017). Harm reduction in the USA: The research perspective and an archive to David Purchase. *Harm Reduction Journal, 26, 14*(1), 51. doi: 10.1186/s12954-017-0178-6

Dishion, T. J., McCord, J., & Poulin, F. (1999). When interventions harm: Peer groups and problem behavior. *American Psychologist, 54*(9), 755–764. https://doi.org/10.1037/0003-066X.54.9.755

Doberstein, C. (2022). "Insite in Vancouver: North America's first supervised injection site," in Evert Lindquist, et al. (eds), *Policy Success in Canada: Cases, Lessons, Challenges*, Oxford, UK: Oxford University Press. https://doi.org/10.1093/oso/9780192897046.003.0004

Drug Enforcement Administration. (December, 16, 2024). *Overdose deaths decline, fentanyl threat looms.* https://www.dea.gov/press-releases/2024/12/16/overdose-deaths-decline-fentanyl-threat-looms

Drug Policy Alliance. (2023, March 22). *Safety first: Real drug education for teens.* Fact Sheet. https://drugpolicy.org/resource/safety-first/

Drug Policy Alliance. (2024, September). *The drug treatment debate: Why accessible and voluntary treatment wins out over forced.* https://drugpolicy.org/wp-content/uploads/2024/09/TheDrugTreatmentDebate_10.30.24-Interactive.pdf

Duster, T. (1970). *The legislation of morality: Law, drugs, and moral judgment.* Free Press: Ann Arbor, MI.

Dylan, E., Kirsch, E., Lippard, T. C. (2002). Early life stress and substance use disorders: The critical role of adolescent substance use, *Pharmacology Biochemistry and Behavior, 215*,173360, ISSN 0091-3057. https://doi.org/10.1016/j.pbb.2022.173360

Education Law Center. (n.d.). *Stopping the school-to-prison pipeline.* https://www.elc-pa.org/stopping-the-school-to-prison-pipeline/

English, A., & Gudeman, R. (2024). *Minor consent and confidentiality: A compendium of state and federal laws.* National Center for Youth Law. https://youthlaw.org/sites/default/files/2024-10/NCYLMinorConsentCompendium2024.pdf

Erikson, E. H. (1950). *Childhood and society.* W. W. Norton & Company.

Erikson, E. H. (1968). *Identity: Youth and crisis.* W. W. Norton & Company.

Erowid. (2025). *DrugsData News – Administrative Pause Explained.* https://www.erowid.org/columns/crew/?p=1378

Evans-Polce, R., Patrick, M., Lanza, S., Miech, R., O'Malley, P., & Johnston, L. (2018). Reasons for vaping among U.S. 12th graders. *Journal of Adolescent Health, 62*(4), 457–462.

Fadus, M. C., Squeglia, L. M., Valadez, E. A. et al. (2019). Adolescent substance use disorder treatment: An update on evidence-based strategies. *Curr Psychiatry Rep*, 21, 96. https://doi.org/10.1007/s11920-019-1086-0

Fair, H., & Walmsley, R. (2021). *World prison population list, 13th edition*. Institute for Crime and Justice Policy Research.

Feldman, N. (November 16, 2020). Safehouse debate in appeals court centers on two sentences in 'crackhouse statute'. WHYY: PBS and NPR affiliate. https://whyy.org/articles/safehouse-debate-in-appeals-court-centers-on-two-sentences-in-crackhouse-statute/

Fleming, T., Barker, A., Ivsins, A., Vakharia, S., & McNeil, R. (2020). Stimulant safe supply: A potential opportunity to respond to the overdose epidemic. *Harm Reduction Journal*, 17, 6–12.

Foote, J., Wilkens, C., Kosanke, N., & Higgs, S. (2014). *Beyond addiction: How science and kindness help people change*. New York: Scribner.

Ford, C. A., English, A., Sigman, G., & the Committee on Adolescence. (2023). Confidentiality in the care of adolescents. *Pediatrics*, 153(5), e2024066326. https://doi.org/10.1542/peds.2024-066326

Friedman, J., & Hadland, S. (2024). The overdose crisis among US adolescents. *The New England Journal of Medicine*, 390(2), 97–100.

Giulini, F., Keenan, E., Killeen, N., & Ivers, J. H. (2022). A systematized review of drug-checking and related considerations for implementation as a harm reduction intervention. *Journal of Psychoactive Drugs*, 55(1), 85–93. https://doi.org/10.1080/02791072.2022.2028203

Godley, S. H., Garner, B. R., Passetti, L. L., Funk, R. R., Dennis, M. L., & Godley, M. D. (2010). Adolescent Community Reinforcement Approach implementation: Fidelity and effectiveness of a performance-based training system. *Journal of Substance Abuse Treatment*, 38(4), 286–295. https://doi.org/10.1016/j.jsat.2010.01.005

Gone, J. P. (2013). Redressing First Nations historical trauma: Theorizing mechanisms for Indigenous culture as mental health treatment. *Transcultural Psychiatry*, 50(5), 683–706.

Greenson, R. R. (1967). *The technique and practice of psychoanalysis* (Vol. 1). International Universities Press.

Groves, M., & Van Sciver, A. (2022). The effectiveness of dialectical behavior therapy for adolescents with substance use disorders: A systematic review. *Children and Youth Services Review*, 139, 106577.

Haidt, J. (2023, February 1). *After Babel*. https://www.afterbabel.com/

Haidt, J. (2024). *The anxious generation: How the great rewiring of childhood is causing an epidemic of mental illness*. Penguin Press.

Haidt, J., & Lukianoff, G. (2021). *The coddling of the American mind: How good intentions and bad ideas are setting up a generation for failure*. Penguin Press.

Harith, S. (1999). Individual risk factors for adolescent substance use. *Drug and Alcohol Dependence*, 55(3), 209–224. https://doi.org/10.1016/S0376-8716(99)00017-4

Harm Reduction Hedgehogs (HRH413). (n.d.). *Home*. https://www.hrh413.org/home

Hart, C. (2013). *High price: A neuroscientist's journey of self-discovery that challenges everything you know about drugs and society*. New York, NY: Harper Perennial.

Hart, C. (2021). *Drug use for grownups*. New York, NY: Penguin Books.

He, J., Yan, X., Wang, R., Zhao, J., Liu, J., Zhou, C., & Zeng, Y. (2022). Does childhood adversity lead to drug addiction in adulthood? A study of serial mediators based on resilience and depression. *Frontiers of Psychiatry*, 18(13), 871459. doi: 10.3389/fpsyt.2022.871459

Herzberg, D. (2020). *Big pharma and the hidden history of addiction in America*. Chicago, IL: University of Chicago Press.

Heyman, G. (2009) *Addiction: A disorder of choice*. Harvard University Press.

Hill, M., Sternberg, A., Suk, H. W., Meier, M. H., & Chassin, L. (2018). The intergenerational transmission of cannabis use: Associations between parental history of cannabis use and cannabis use disorder, low positive parenting, and offspring cannabis use. *Psychology of Addictive Behaviors*, 32(1), 93–103. https://doi.org/10.1037/adb0000333

Hogue, A., Henderson, C. E., Becker, S. J., & Knight, D. K. (2014). Evidence base on outpatient behavioral treatments for adolescent substance use, 2014–2017: Outcomes, treatment delivery, and promising directions. *Journal of Clinical Child & Adolescent Psychology*, *43*(4), 529–549.

Human Rights Watch. (2025). *Punishment and prejudice: Racial disparities and the War on Drugs*. https://www.hrw.org/legacy/campaigns/drugs/war/key-facts.htm

Hunt, N. (2010). *A review of the evidence-base for harm reduction approaches to drug use*. International Harm Reduction Association. https://hri.global/files/2010/05/31/HIVTop50Documents11.pdf

Hussong, A. M., Ennett, S. T., Cox, M. J., & Haroon, M. (2017). A systematic review of the unique prospective association of negative affect symptoms and adolescent substance use controlling for externalizing symptoms. *Psychology of Addictive Behaviors*, *31*(2), 137–147.

Inciardi, J. A., & Harrison, L. D. (2000). *Harm reduction: National and international perspectives*. Sage Publications.

International Drug Policy Consortium. (2020). Taking back what ours! An oral history of the movement of people who use drugs. https://idpc.net/news/2020/08/taking-back-what-s-ours-an-oral-history-of-the-movement-of-people-who-use-drugs

Janis, I. L., & Mann, L. (1977). *Decision making: A psychological analysis of conflict, choice, and commitment*. Free Press.

Jenkins, E., Slemon, A., & Haines-Saah, R. (2017). Developing harm reduction in the context of youth substance use: Insights from a multi-site qualitative analysis of young people's harm minimization strategies. *Harm Reduction Journal*, *14*, 53–64.

Jensen, C. D., Cushing, C. C., Aylward, B. S., Craig, J. T., Sorell, D. M., & Steele, R. G. (2011). Effectiveness of motivational interviewing interventions for adolescent substance use behavior change: A meta-analytic review. *Journal of Consulting and Clinical Psychology*, *79*(4), 433–440. https://doi.org/10.1037/a0023992

Miech, R. A., Johnston, L. D., Patrick, M. E., & O'Malley, P. M. (2025). Monitoring the future national survey results on drug use, 1975–2024: Overview and detailed results for secondary school students. *Monitoring the Future Monograph Series*. Institute for Social Research, University of Michigan. https://monitoringthefuture.org/results/annual-reports/

Jones, J. (April 29th, 2021). *America's forgotten history of supervised opiate injection*. Undark. https://undark.org/2021/04/29/forgotten-history-supervised-injection/

Kandel, D., Yamaguchi, K., & Chen, K. (1992). Stages of progression in drug involvement from adolescence to adulthood: Further evidence for the gateway theory. *Journal of Studies on Alcohol*, *53*(5), 447–457.

Kellogg, S. (2003). On "gradualism" and the building of the harm reduction-abstinence continuum. *Journal of Substance Abuse Treatment*, *25*, 241–247.

Kellogg, S. (2013). *Transformational chairwork: Using psychotherapeutic dialogues in clinical practice*. Rowman & Littlefield.

Kellogg, S. (2024). *With love and intensity: Some reflections on chairwork, harm reduction psychotherapy, and the treatment of addictions*. Chairwork Psychotherapy Initiative.

Kellogg, S., & Tatarsky, A. (2012) Re-envisioning addiction treatment: A six-point plan. *Alcoholism Treatment Quarterly*, *30*(1), 109–128.

Kerr, T., Mitra, S., Kennedy, M.C. et al. (2017). Supervised injection facilities in Canada: past, present, and future. *Harm Reduction Journal*, *14*(28). https://doi.org/10.1186/s12954-017-0154-1

Khantzian, E. J. (1997). The self-medication hypothesis of substance use disorders: A reconsideration and recent applications. *Harvard Review of Psychiatry*, *4*(5), 231–244.

Kidorf, M., King, V. L., Peirce, J., Kolodner, K., & Brooner, R. K. (2011). Benefits of concurrent syringe exchange and substance abuse treatment participation. *Journal of Substance Abuse Treatment*, *40*(3), 265–271. doi: 10.1016/j.jsat.2010.11.011

Kim, B. K., Oesterle, S., Catalano, R., & Hawkins, J. (2015). Change in protective factors across adolescent development. *Journal of Applied Developmental Psychology*, *40*, 26–37.

Kimball, C., & Grawert, A. (2021). *Collateral consequences and the enduring nature of punishment*. Brennan Center for Justice. https://www.brennancenter.org/our-work/analysis-opinion/collateral-consequences-and-enduring-nature-punishment

King, C., Beetham, T., Smith, N., Englander, H., Hadland, S. E., Bagley, S. M., & Korthuis, P. T. (2023). Treatments used among adolescent residential addiction treatment facilities in the US, 2022. *JAMA, 329*(22), 1983–1985. https://doi.org/10.1001/jama.2023.6266

King, V., Mrug, S., & Windle, M. (2022). Predictors of motives for marijuana use in African American adolescents and emerging adults. *Journal of Ethnicity in Substance Abuse, 21*(1), 3–21.

Kirsch, D. E., & Lippard, E. T. C. (2022). Early life stress and substance use disorders: The critical role of adolescent substance use. *Pharmacology Biochemistry and Behavior, 215*, 173360. https://doi.org/10.1016/j.pbb.2022.173360

Kleinig, J. (2008). The ethics of harm reduction. *Substance Use & Misuse, 43*(1), 1–16. https://doi.org/10.1080/10826080701690680

Kleinig, J. (2015). Ready for retirement: The gateway drug hypothesis. *Substance Use and Misuse, early online, 1–5*. doi: 10.3109/10826084.2015.1007679

Kluckow, R., & Zeng, Z. (2022). *Correctional populations of the United States*. Bureau of Justice Statistics.

Kral, A., Lambdin, B., Wenger, L., & Davidson, P. (2020). Correspondence: Evaluation of an unsanctioned safe consumption site in the United States. *New England Journal of Medicine, 383*, 589–590. doi: 10.1056/NEJMc2015435

Kristen, L., Paquette, L. A., Pannella, W., Catriona, M., Wilkey, K. N., Ferreira, L. R., & Donegan, W. (2019). A framework for integrating young peers in recovery into adolescent substance use prevention and early intervention, *Addictive Behaviors, 99*. https://doi.org/10.1016/j.addbeh.2019.106080

Kumar, R., O'Malley, P., Johnston, L., & Laetz, V. (2013). Alcohol, Tobacco, and Other Drug Use Prevention Programs in U.S. Schools: A Descriptive Summary *Prev Sci.* 2013 Dec; *14*(6): 581–592. doi: 10.1007/s11121-012-0340-z

Larimer, M., Lee, C., Kilmer, J., Fabiano, P., Stark, C., Geisner, I., ... Neighbors, C. (2007). Personalized mailed feedback for college drinking prevention: A randomized clinical trial. *Journal of Consulting and Clinical Psychology, 75*(2), 285–293.

Leonard, N. (April 23, 2024). Federal judge dismisses Philadelphia Safehouse case, which sought a legal pathway for supervised injection sites. WHYY: PBS and NPR affiliate. https://whyy.org/articles/philadelphia-safehouse-case-supervised-injection-judge-dismisses/

Lessin, B. (2023a). *Helping Teens with substance use problems: Why I changed my approach*. https://www.barrylessin.com/helping-teens-with-substance-use-problems-why-i-changed-my-approach

Lessin, B. (May 18, 2023b). *Teenagers pathologized by traditional addiction treatment*. https://filtermag.org/addiction-treatment-pathologize-teenagers/

Levengood, T. W., Yoon, G. H., Davoust, M.J., Ogden, S. N., Marshall, B. D. L., Cahill, S. R., & Bazzi, A. R. (2021). Supervised injection facilities as harm reduction: A systematic review. *American Journal of Preventive Medicine, 61*(5), 738–749. doi: 10.1016/j.amepre.2021.04.017

Levine, B. (2013, July 31). *Why the rise of mental illness? Pathologizing normal, adverse drug effects, and a peculiar rebellion*. https://www.madinamerica.com/2013/07/why-the-dramatic-rise-of-mental-illness-diseasing-normal-behaviors-drug-adverse-effects-and-a-peculiar-rebellion/

Linehan, M. M. (2015). *DBT skills training manual* (2nd ed.). Guilford Press.

Logan, D., & Marlatt, G. A. (2010). Harm reduction therapy: A practice-friendly review of research. *Journal of Clinical Psychology, 66*(2): 201–214.

Maccoby, E. E., & Martin, J. A. (1983). Socialization in the context of the family: Parent-child interaction. In P. H. Mussen (Ed.), *Handbook of child psychology* (Vol. 4, pp. 1–101). New York: Wiley.

Marlatt, G. A., & Donovan, D. M. (Eds.). (2005). *Relapse prevention: Maintenance strategies in the treatment of addictive behaviors* (2nd ed.). Guilford Press.

Marlatt, G. A., Larimer, M. E., & Witkiewitz, K. (2012). *Harm reduction: Pragmatic strategies for managing high-risk behaviors* (2nd ed.). Guilford Press.

Marlatt, G. A. (1996). Harm reduction: Come as you are. *Addictive Behaviors, 21*(6), 779–788.

Marlatt, G. A., & Witkiewitz, K. (2002). Harm reduction approaches to alcohol use: Health promotion, prevention and treatment. *Addictive Behaviors, 27*, 867–886.

Marlatt, G. A., & Witkiewitz, K. (2010). Update on harm reduction intervention policy and research. *Annual Review of Clinical Psychology*, *6*, 591–606.

Maslow, A. H. (1970). *Motivation and personality* (2nd ed.). Harper & Row.

Maté, G. (2010). *In the realm of hungry ghosts: Close encounters with addiction*. North Atlantic Books.

Matusow, H., Dickman, S. L., Rich, J. D., Fong, C., Dumont, D. M., Hardin, C., ... & Rosenblum, A. (2013). Medication-assisted treatment in U.S. drug courts: Results from a nationwide survey of availability, barriers and attitudes. *Journal of Substance Abuse Treatment*, *44*(5), 473–480. https://doi.org/10.1016/j.jsat.2012.10.004

Mauer, M., Potler, C., & Wolf, W. (1999). *Gender and justice: Women, drugs and sentencing policy*. The Sentencing Project. https://static.prisonpolicy.org/scans/sp/genderandjustice.pdf

McGinnis, H. A., & Wright, A. W. (2023). Adoption and child health and psychosocial well-being. In B. Halpern-Felsher (Ed.), *Encyclopedia of child and adolescent health* (1st Edition), Academic Press, pp. 582–598. https://doi.org/10.1016/B978-0-12-818872-9.00115-1

Merlin, A., O'Malley, P., Schulenberg, J., Bachman, J., & Johnston, L. (2004). Substance use among adults 35 years of age: Prevalence, adulthood predictors, and impact of adolescent substance use. *American Journal of Public Health*, *94*(1), 96–102.

Meyers, R. J. (n.d.-a). *Community Reinforcement Training*. https://www.robertjmeyersphd.com/craft-cra-acra-professional-training

Meyers, R. J. (n.d.-b). *Self-guided online CRAFT Training Program*. We The Village. https://www.robertjmeyersphd.com/training/self-guided-online-craft-training-program

Meyers, R. J., Miller, W. R., Smith, J. E., & Tonigan, J. S. (2002). A randomized trial of two methods for engaging treatment-refusing drug users through concerned significant others. *Journal of Consulting and Clinical Psychology*, *70*(5), 1182–1185. https://doi.org/10.1037/0022-006X.70.5.1182

Miller, W. R., & Rollnick, S. (1991). *Motivational interviewing: Preparing people to change addictive behavior*. Guilford Press.

Miller, W. R., & Rollnick, S. (2012). *Motivational Interviewing: Helping people change* (3rd ed.). Guilford Press.

Moss, H. B., Chen, C. M., &Yi, H.-Y. (2014). Early adolescent patterns of alcohol, cigarettes, and marijuana polysubstance use and young adult substance use outcomes in a nationally representative sample, *Drug and Alcohol Dependence*, *136*, 51–62. https://doi.org/10.1016/j.drugalcdep.2013.12.011

Musto, D. (1999). *The American disease: The origins of narcotics control*. Oxford, UK: Oxford University Press.

Najavits, L. M. (2002). *Seeking safety: A treatment manual for PTSD and substance abuse*. Guilford Press.

Najavits, L. M. (2022). *Creating change: A past-focused treatment for trauma and addiction*. Guilford Press.

National Alliance on Mental Illness. (n.d.). https://www.nami.org/

National Association of Criminal Defense Lawyers. (November 29, 2022). *Race and the War on Drugs*. https://www.nacdl.org/Content/Race-and-the-War-on-Drugs

National Harm Reduction Coalition (n.d.-a). *Online training institute*. https://harmreduction.org/our-work/training-capacity-building/online-training-institute/

National Harm Reduction Coalition (n.d.-b). *Resource center*. https://harmreduction.org/resource-center/

National Harm Reduction Coalition, (2024). https://harmreduction.org/movement/evolution/

Nawi, A. M., Ismail, R., Ibrahim, F., Jalani, F. A., & Abdullah, N. (2021). Family and peer influences on adolescent drug abuse: A qualitative study among Malaysian adolescents. *BMC Public Health*, *21*(1), Article 2235. https://doi.org/10.1186/s12889-021-11906-2

Neighbors, C., Larimer, M., Lostutter, T., & Woods, B. (2006). Harm reduction and individually focused alcohol prevention. *International Journal of Drug Policy*, *17*(4), 304–309.

Nellis, A. (2021). *The color of justice: Racial and ethnic disparities in state prisons*. The Sentencing Project.

Network for Public Health Law. (2024, October). *Legal interventions to reduce overdose mortality: Naloxone access and Good Samaritan laws.* https://www.networkforphl.org/resources/legal-interventions-to-reduce-overdose-mortality-naloxone-access-and-good-samaritan-laws/

O'Hare, P. (2007). Merseyside, the first harm reduction conferences, and the early history of harm reduction. *International Journal of Drug Policy, 18,* 141–144.

Olsoon, C., Bond, L., Burns, J., Vella-Brodrick, D., & Sawyer, S. (2003). Adolescent resilience: A concept analysis. *Journal of Adolescence, 26,* 1–11.

Otten, R., Mun, C. J., Shaw, D. S., Wilson, M. N., & Dishion, T. J. (2019). A developmental cascade model for early adolescent-onset substance use: the role of early childhood stress. *Addiction, 114,* 326–334. https://doi.org/10.1111/add.14452

Paquette, C. E., Daughters, S. B., & Witkiewitz, K. (2022). Expanding the continuum of substance use disorder treatment: Nonabstinence approaches. *Clinical Psychology Review, 91,* 102110. https://doi.org/10.1016/j.cpr.2021.102110

Paquette, K. L., Winn, L. A. P., Wilkey, C. M., Ferreira, K. N., & Donegan, L. R. W. (2019). A framework for integrating young peers in recovery into adolescent substance use prevention and early intervention. *Addictive Behaviors, 99,* 106080. https://doi.org/10.1016/j.addbeh.2019.106080

Partnership to End Addiction. (n.d.). *Drugfree.org.* https://drugfree.org

Paterson, B., & Panessa, C. (2008). Engagement as an ethical imperative in harm reduction involving at-risk youth. International Journal of Drug Policy, 19(1), 24–32. doi: 10.1016/j.drugpo.2007.11.007

Patrick, M., Miech, R., Carlier, C., O'Malley, P., Johnston, L., & Schulenberg, J. (2016). Self-reported reasons for vaping among 8th, 10th, and 12th graders in the US: Nationally-representative results. *Drug and Alcohol Dependence, 165,* 275–278.

Patrick, M., Terry-McElrath, Y., Arterberry, B., & Miech, R. (2024). Reasons for Vaping among US adolescents. *Pediatrics, 154*(6), e2024067856.

Peele, S. (1998). The results for drug policy reform goals of shifting from interdiction/punishment to treatment. *International Journal of Drug Policy, 9,* 43–56.

Peele, S. (2007.) *Addiction proof your child: A realistic approach to preventing drug, alcohol, and other dependencies.* New York: Harmony.

Peele, S., & Brodsky, A. (1975). *Love and addiction.* New American Library.

Peele, S., & Brodsky, A. (1991). *The truth about addiction and recovery: The life process program for outgrowing destructive habits.* Simon & Schuster.

Peltz, J. (March 9, 2022). *A look inside the 1st official safe injection sites in the U.S.* PBS News. https://www.pbs.org/newshour/health/a-look-inside-the-1st-official-safe-injection-sites-in-u-s

Platt, L., Minozzi, S., Reed, J., Vickerman, P., Hagan, H., French, C., … Hickman, M. (2018). Needle and syringe programmes and opioid substitution therapy for preventing HCV transmission among people who inject drugs: findings from a Cochrane Review and meta-analysis. *Addiction, 113*(3), 545–563.

Post, B. C., & Wade, N. G. (2009). Religion and spirituality in psychotherapy: A practice-friendly review of research. *Journal of Clinical Psychology, 65*(2), 131–146. https://doi.org/10.1002/jclp.20563

Potier, C., Laprévote, V., Dubois-Arber, F., Cottencin, O., & Rolland, B. (2014). Supervised injection services: what has been demonstrated? A systematic literature review. *Drug and Alcohol Dependence, 1*(145), 48–68. doi: 10.1016/j.drugalcdep.2014.10.012

Prochaska, J. O., & DiClemente, C. C. (1983). Stages and processes of self-change of smoking: Toward an integrative model of change. *Journal of Consulting and Clinical Psychology, 51*(3), 390–395. https://doi.org/10.1037/0022-006X.51.3.390

Pure Food and Drug Act. (1906). https://www.fda.gov/about-fda/changes-science-law-and-regulatory-authorities/part-i-1906-food-and-drugs-act-and-its-enforcement

Rathus, J. H., & Miller, A. L. (2002). *Dialectical behavior therapy adapted for adolescents.* New Harbinger Publications.

Richards, D., Pearson, M., & Witkiewitz, K. (2021). Understanding alcohol harm reduction behaviors from the perspective of self-determination theory: A research agenda. *Addiction Research Theory, 29*(5), 392–397.

Rigter, H., Henderson, C., Pelc, I., Tossman, P., Phan, O., Hendricks, V., ... Lowe, C. (2013). Multidimensional family therapy lowers the rate of cannabis dependence in adolescents: A randomised controlled trial in Western European outpatient settings. *Drug and Alcohol Dependence*, *130*, 85–93.

Robey, J., Massoglia, M., & Light, M. (2023). *A generational shift: Race and the declining lifetime risk of imprisonment*. Demography. https://doi.org/10.1215/00703370-10863378

Rogers, C. R. (1961). *On becoming a person: A therapist's view of psychotherapy*. Boston: Houghton Mifflin.

Rotgers, F. (2022). My brain disease made me do it: Bioethical implications of the Brain Disease Model of Addiction. In N. Heather, M. Field, A. C. Moss, & S. Satel (Eds.), *Evaluating the brain disease model of addiction* (pp. 217–230). Routledge.

Rotgers, F., & Davis, B. A. (2006). *Treating alcohol problems*. Wiley.

Ryan, C., Huebner, D., Diaz, R. M., & Sanchez, J. (2009). Family rejection as a predictor of negative health outcomes in white and Latino lesbian, gay, and bisexual young adults. *Pediatrics*, *123*(1), 346–352.

SAMHSA. (2021). *Medications for opioid use disorder (MOUD) treatment improvement protocol (TIP) 63*. Substance Abuse and Mental Health Services Administration.

SAMHSA. (2023). *National Survey on Drug Use and Health*. Retrieved March 2025 from https://www.samhsa.gov/data/data-we-collect/nsduh-national-survey-drug-use-and-health/datafiles

Satir, V. (1964). *Conjoint family therapy*. Palo Alto, CA: Science and Behavior Books,

Sawangjit, R., Khan, T. M., & Chaiyakunapruk, N. (2017). Effectiveness of pharmacy-based needle/syringe exchange programme for people who inject drugs: A systematic review and meta-analysis. *Addiction*, *112*(2), 236–247.

Schwartz, S. J., Unger, J. B., Zamboanga, B. L., & Szapocznik, J. (2010). Rethinking the concept of acculturation: Implications for theory and research. *American Psychologist*, *65*(4), 237–251.

Schwebel, F., Richards, D., Pearson, M., & Witikiewitz, K. (2024). Initial psychometric testing of the Harm Reduction Self-Efficacy Scale (HRSES). *Addiction Research Theory*, *32*(6), 392–399.

Secades-Villa, R., Garcia-Rodríguez, O., Jin, C., Wang, S., & Blanco, C. (2014). Probability and predictors of the cannabis gateway effect: A national study. *International Journal of Drug Policy*. http://dx.doi.org/10.1016/j.drugpo.2014.07.011

Shrier, L. A., Harris, S. K., Kurland, M., & Knight, J. R. (June 2003). Substance use problems and associated psychiatric symptoms among adolescents in primary care. *Pediatrics*, *111*(6), e699–e705. doi: 10.1542/peds.111.6.e699

Simon, C., Brothers, S., Strichartz, K., Coulter, A., Voyles, N., Herdlein, A., & Vincent, L. (2021). We are the researched, the researchers, and the discounted: The experiences of drug user activists as researchers. *International Journal of Drug Policy*, *98*, 103364. doi: 10.1016/j.drugpo.2021.103364

Skinner-Osei, P., & Levenson, J. S. (2018). Trauma-informed services for children with incarcerated parents. *Journal of Family Social Work*, *21*(4–5), 421–437. https://doi.org/10.1080/10522158.2018.1499064

Smith, D. C., Godley, S. H., Godley, M. D., & Dennis, M. L. (2011). Adolescent Community Reinforcement Approach (A-CRA) outcomes differ among emerging adults and adolescents. *Journal of Substance Abuse Treatment*, *41*(4), 422–430. https://doi.org/10.1016/j.jsat.2011.05.003

Smith, J. E., & Meyers, R. J. (2023). *The CRAFT Treatment Manual for Substance Use Problems: Working with family members*. Guilford Press.

Sousa, M. D. (2021). Procedural due process, drug courts, and loss of liberty sanctions. *New York University Journal of Law & Liberty*, *14*(3), 733–799.

St. Arnaud, K. O. (2021). Toward a positive psychology of psychoactive drug use. *Drugs: Education, Prevention and Policy*, *30*(1), 81–94. https://doi.org/10.1080/09687637.2021.2002816

Staff, J., Schulenberg, J., Maslowsky, J., Bachman, J., O'Malley, P., Maggs, J., & Johnston, L. (2010). Substance use changes and social role transitions: Proximal developmental effects on ongoing trajectories from late adolescence through early adulthood. *Developmental Psychopathology*, *22*(4), 917–932.

Steiker, L. (2008). Making drug and alcohol prevention relevant. *Family and Community Health, 32*(Supplement 1), S52–S60.

Steinberg, L. (2005). *The Ten Basic Principles of Good Parenting*. Simon & Schuster.

Steinberg, L. (2014). *Age of opportunity: Lessons from the new science of adolescence*. Houghton Mifflin Harcourt.

Stockings, E., Hall, W., Lynskey, M., Morley, K., Reavley, N., Stang, J., ... Degenhardt, L. (2016). Substance use in young people. *Lancet Psychiatry, 3*, 280–296.

Stockwell, T., Toumbourou, J., Letcher, P., Smart, D., Sanson, A., & Bond, L. (2004). Risk and protection factors for different intensities of adolescent substance use: When does the Prevention Paradox apply? *Drug and Alcohol Review, 23*, 67–77.

Stout, D. D. (2009). *Coming to harm reduction kicking & screaming: Looking for harm reduction in a 12-step world*. AuthorHouse.

Substance Abuse and Mental Health Services Administration. (2020). *TIP 65: Counseling approaches to promote recovery from substance use disorders* (Publication No. PEP20-02-01-004). U.S. Department of Health and Human Services. https://library.samhsa.gov/sites/default/files/pep20-02-01-004.pdf

Sue, D. W., Sue, D., Neville, H. A., & Smith, L. (2019). *Counseling the culturally diverse: Theory and practice* (8th ed.). John Wiley & Sons.

Sugie, N. (2015). Chilling effects: Diminished political participation among partners of formerly incarcerated men. Social Problems, *62*(4), 550–571.

Szalavitz, M. (2006). *Help at any cost: How the troubled-teen industry cons parents and hurts kids*. Riverhead Books

Szalavitz, M. (2016). *Unbroken brain: A revolutionary new way of understanding addiction*. St. Martin's Press.

Taifa, N. (May 10, 2021). *Race, mass incarceration, and the disastrous War on Drugs*. Brennan Center. https://www.brennancenter.org/our-work/analysis-opinion/race-mass-incarceration-and-disastrous-war-drugs

Tanner-Smith, E. E., Wilson, S. J., & Lipsey, M. W. (2013). The comparative effectiveness of outpatient treatment for adolescent substance abuse: A meta-analysis. *Journal of Substance Abuse Treatment, 44*(2), 145–158. https://doi.org/10.1016/j.jsat.2012.05.006

Tapert, S., Aarons, G., Sedlar, G., & Brown, S. (2001). Adolescent substance use and sexual risk-taking behavior. *Journal of Adolescent Health, 28*, 181–189.

Tatarsky, A. (2002). *Harm reduction psychotherapy: A new treatment for drug and alcohol problems*. Jason Aronson, Inc.

Tatarsky, A. (2003). Harm reduction psychotherapy: Extending the reach of traditional substance use treatment. *Journal of Substance Abuse Treatment, 25*(4), 249–256. https://doi.org/10.1016/S0740-5472(03)00085-0

Tatarsky, A., & Kellogg, S. H. (2010). Integrative harm reduction psychotherapy: A six-session treatment for high-risk drug and alcohol users. *Journal of Clinical Psychology, 66*(2), 137–146. https://doi.org/10.1002/jclp.20626

Text - S.2633 - 107th Congress. (2001-2002): RAVE Act. (2002, October 9). https://www.congress.gov/bill/107th-congress/senate-bill/2633/text

The Seven Challenges. n.d. *Overview for Adolescents*. https://www.sevenchallenges.com/overview/for-adolescents/

Thorton, M. (1991). *Alcohol prohibition was a failure. Policy Analysis, 157*. Cato Institute. https://www.cato.org/policy-analysis/alcohol-prohibition-was-failure?fbclid=IwAR3Spf2-h4D8lI6j57iguopvHoLA3NQLl4b4SIvd7AtqEJVnYi-3UxYxI8Y

Toumbourou, J., Gregg, M., Shortt, A., Hutchinson, D., & Slaviero, T. (2013). Reduction of adolescent alcohol use through family-school intervention: A randomized trial. *Journal of Adolescent Health, 53*, 778–784.

Toumbourou, J., Stockwell, T., Neighbors, C., Marlatt, G., Sturge, J., & Rehm, J. (2007). Interventions to reduce harm associated with adolescent substance use. *Lancet, 369*, 1391–1401.

Toumbourou, J., Williams, I., Snow, P., & White, V. (2003). Adolescent alcohol-use trajectories in the transition from high school. *Drug and Alcohol Review, 22*, 111–116.

Trickett, E. J., & Jones, C. J. (2007). Adolescent culture and formal structure in multicultural community-based programs. *American Journal of Community Psychology*, *39*(1–2), 31–42.

Twenge, J. M., Haidt, J., Lozano, J., & Cummins, K. M. (2022). Specification curve analysis shows that social media use is linked to poor mental health, especially among girls. *Acta Psychologica*, *224*, 103512. https://doi.org/10.1016/j.actpsy.2022.103512

US Food and Drug Administration (2025). Results from the Annual National Youth Tobacco Survey. https://www.fda.gov/tobacco-products/youth-and-tobacco/results-annual-national-youth-tobacco-survey?utm_source=chatgpt.com

Utah, S.B. 152, Social Media Regulation Act, 2023 Gen. Sess. (Utah 2023). https://le.utah.gov/~2023/bills/static/SB0152.html

Vakharia, S. (2024). *The harm reduction gap*. Routledge.

Vakharia, S. P., & Little, J. (2017). Starting where the client is: Harm reduction guidelines for clinical social work practice. *Clinical Social Work Journal*, *45*(1), 65–76. https://doi.org/10.1007/s10615-016-0584-3

Van Dam, T, (2008). *Users unite: A brief overview about the drug user movement*. Amsterdam, Netherlands: Foundation Regenboog AMOC. https://www.aidsactioneurope.org/sites/default/files/1103-0_0.pdf

van der Kolk, B. A. (2014). *The body keeps the score: Brain, mind, and body in the healing of trauma*. New York: Viking.

Van Ryzin, M. J., Fosco, G. M., & Dishion, T. J. (2012). Family and peer predictors of substance use from early adolescence to early adulthood: An 11-year prospective analysis, *Addictive Behaviors*, *37*(12), 1314–1324. https://doi.org/10.1016/j.addbeh.2012.06.020

Vermont Department of Health. (2024). *Vermont Overdose Prevention Center Operating Guidelines*. https://www.healthvermont.gov/sites/default/files/document/dsu-overdose-prevention-center-guidelines.pdf

Volkow, N. D., & Koob, G. F. (2015). Brain disease model of addiction: Why is it so controversial? *The Lancet Psychiatry*, *2*(8), 677–679. https://doi.org/10.1016/S2215-0366(15)00236-9

Volkow, N. D., Frieden, T. R., Hyde, P. S., & Cha, S. S. (2014). Medication-assisted therapies – tackling the opioid-overdose epidemic. *New England Journal of Medicine*, *370*(22), 2063–2066. https://doi.org/10.1056/NEJMp1402780

Wait Until 8th. (n.d.). Join the movement. https://www.waituntil8th.org/

Wald, J., & Losen, D. J. (2023). Defining and redirecting a school-to-prison pipeline. New directions for youth development. *Dignity in Schools Campaign*, (99), 9–15. https://dignityinschools.org/

Wang, P., Williams, R., Chen, W., Wang, F., Shamout, M., Tanz, L., … Kumagai, K. (2024). Chemical composition of electronic vaping products from school grounds in California, *Nicotine & Tobacco Research*, *26*(8), 991–998. https://doi.org/10.1093/ntr/ntae042

Weil, A. (2004). *The natural mind: A new way of looking at drugs and the higher consciousness* (Rev. ed.). Houghton Mifflin Harcourt.

Welsh, J., Dopp, A., Durham, R., Sitar, S., Passetti, L., Hunter, S., … Winters, K. (2025). Narrative review: Revised principles and practice recommendations for adolescent substance use treatment and policy. *Journal of the American Academy for Adolescent Psychiatry*, *64*(2), 123–142.

Welsh, J., Mataczynski, M., Sarvey, D., & Zoltani, J. (2020). Management of complex co-occurring psychiatric disorders and high-risk behavior in adolescence. *Focus*, *18*, 139–149.

White, W. L. (2014). *Slaying the dragon: The history of addiction treatment and recovery in America*. Chestnut Health Systems/Lighthouse Institute.

Whiteside, U., Cronce, J., Pederson, E., & Larimer, M. (2010). Brief motivational feedback for college students and adolescents: A harm reduction approach. *Journal of Clinical Psychology*, *66*(2), 150–163.

Wicklund, R. A. (1974). *Freedom and reactance*. Lawrence Erlbaum Associates.

Wild, T. C., et al. (2018). Mandatory addiction treatment: Ethical considerations and the harm reduction perspective. *Substance Abuse Treatment, Prevention, and Policy*, *13*(1), 1–10.

Wodak, A. (2007). Ethics and drug policy. *Psychiatry*, *6*(2), 59–62.

Zinberg, N. (1986). *Drug, set, and setting: The basis for controlled intoxicant use*. Yale University Press.

Index

Note: Locators in **bold** indicate tables and in ***bold-italics*** boxes.

abstinence focus, mutual aid groups 7–8
acculturation 71
A-CRA (Adolescent Community Reinforcement Approach) 133–134
The Age of Opportunity (Steinberg) 73
Adderall 21, 37, 91, 92, 100, 140
addiction: authoritative parenting approach 82–83; as complex biopsychosocial phenomenon 88–90; definition (DSM-5) 93; drug use vs addiction 1; HRT model 51–52, 63, 89–90; medicalization and disease model narrative *43*, 50, 88–89; medical/spiritual models (AA, NA) 7–8, *42*, 88; vs. physical dependence 93–94; prohibition-based treatment myths 46–49; and trauma 115, 116
adolescent developmental arc and substance use 72–79; adolescent brain plasticity 3, 29, 30, 45, 75–76, 77, 148; cognitive development and moral reasoning 79; early adolescence *74*; emotional and stress-related factors 78; family and environmental factors 79; identity formation and autonomy 77–78, 149; late adolescence *75*; middle adolescence *74–75*; peer influence and social development 78; risk taking, impulsivity 77, 149
age of onset, initiation 25–26, 30, 31, 45, 148; *see also* Gateway Theory
Age-Appropriate Design Code, California 84
AIDS 5, 8
Ainsworth, Mary 119
Al-Anon/Nar-Anon Facilitation (ANF) 44, 121, 134
alcohol: abstinence focus 7–8, 16; addiction treatment models 88–89; gateway theory 25–26; HRT programs, implementation and acceptance 32–34; prevalence, alcohol abuse/dependence and treatment 23–24, **23**; prevalence, use, use pattern 20–22, **22–23**, 24, 90–92; prohibition 16, *42*; safe use continuum **95**; unsafe supply, illegal 36; youth education, information 36

alcohol, early use harm potential and outcome 2–3, 26–30; adolescent presentation 27–28; physical risks 28–29; psychological risks 29–30
Alcoholics Anonymous (AA) 7–8, *42*, 88
Alexander, Bruce 88
all or nothing (abstinence-only) narrative 7–8, *43*, 88
"All use is abuse" approach 2, 7, 10, 22, 24, 30, 32, 38, 147, 148
American Foundation for AIDS Research (amFAR) 12
amphetamine 21, **22**, **24**
Amsterdam syringe access program 12
Anti-Drug Abuse Act (1986) 35
attachment theory and pattern 119, 150
authoritarian parenting *80*, 81
authoritative parenting 44, 73, 74, *80*, 81–83, 84–85, 121, 149
autonomy 57, 63, 65, 66–67, *68–69*, 76–77, 84, 102–103, *124–127*, 149

Baumrind, Diane 79–80, *80*
"Being ready" concept 47–48
Bigg, Dan 90
Black people 9, 35, 46, 70; *see also* racism
The Body Keeps the Score (van der Kolk) 117
Bond, L. 32
brain development/plasticity and substance use 3, 29, 30, 45, 75–76, 77, 148
Brehm, J. W. 45
Brief Alcohol Screening and Intervention for College Students (BASICS) 34
Bryant, A. 32

caffeine 7
cannabis: Cannabis Use Disorder (CUD) 23–24, **24**, 37; exercises 135–137, 137, 138, 140, 141–143; gateway theory 25, 46, 49; habit forming qualities 28; Harm Reduction Psychotherapy (Denning and Little), example 118;

IDEA framework, case example 107–110; medical consumption 12, 37–38; Multi-Dimensional Family Therapy (MDFT 31; obtainability 18; parental, working with, CRAFT examples *124–126*, 127–128, 130–133; parental use impact 35–37; prevalence, consumption patterns 18, 20, *20*, 23, 27, 90–93; prohibition, legalisation, de-stigmatization 17, 18, 28, 35–37, 135–137; risks (physical, psychological) 25; *Seeking Safety* treatment, example 117; THC 28–29, 37; use purposes 101, 102, 104, 117; vaping 22, **23**
Centers for Disease Control (CDC) 16
cigarettes 22–23, **22–24**; *see also* tobacco
cocaine **22, 24**, 35, 93, 101–102
Cognitive Behavioral Therapy (CBT) 52, 110, 112, 113–114, 116, 134, 153
cognitive development: adolescent developmental arc phases *74–75*; deficit mitigation 79; early substance use impact 29; and moral reasoning 79; *see also* brain development/plasticity
collateral sanctions 1, 6, 9, 34, 35
Comas-Díaz, Lillian 70
community: community connections and strengths 70–71; community driven research (CDR) 14, 59; Community Reinforcement and Family Training 120–133; *see also* CRAFT (Community Reinforcement and Family Training); community trauma 35, 70; community-based participatory research (CBPR) 15; community-based/including programs, initiatives 33, 44, 46, 64; drug user's unions 15, 148; substance-using (support, advocacy) 5, 8, 11–12, 14–15, 33
confidentiality 67, *68*, 69
crack **22**, 35
CRAFT (Community Reinforcement and Family Training) 119–121, *122–123*, *124–127*, 152–153
Creating Change treatment 116
criminalization, drug use 1, 8–9; Anti-Drug Abuse Act (1986) 35; concept/narrative, consequences 34–35, 42, 66, 147, 148; courts as gatekeeper narrative *43*; "drug misuse" vs. "drug abuse" 50; family, parenting impact 44–45; gateway theory argument 17; Harrison Narcotics Act (1914) 6; Merseyside (UK) harm reduction vs criminalization approach 5–7; racism, sexism, poverty factors on 9, 35, 46, 66; RAVE Act 16, 28; school, community impact (school-to-prison pipeline) 45–46; War on Drugs 2, 6, 35, 39, *41–43*, 52, 66, 132, 148
cultural contexts and expectations 63, 65, 71–72, 78, *100*, 101
cultural responsiveness 44, 69–72, 70, 71, 149

Dance Safe 16
D.A.R.E. era 25, 36
Decisional Balance 102–104, **104**, 108, 109, 111–112
Denning, Pat 51–52, 55–56, 57–58, 59, 60, 94, 97–98, 115, 118–119
Dialectical Behavior Therapy (DBT) / Dialectical Behavior Therapy for Adolescents (DBT-A) 52, 110, 114, 116
dialectical nature, harm reduction psychotherapy 55, 57–58, 149
Drug, Set, Setting model (Zinberg) 51, 52–53, 97–98, 100–102, *100*, 105
drug checking, substance safety 16, 28, 33, 35, 148
Drug Enforcement Administration (DEA) 16, 102
drug policy: access to evidence-based care 40–41, 50; adolescent overdose risk 38–40; language and communication impact 16, 49–50; narratives and substance use perception/treatment 40–41; prohibition-based, family/parenting impact 44–45; prohibition-based, school/community impact 44–45; prohibition-based myths 46–49
Drug Policy Alliance 36, 90
drug user's unions 15, 148

e-cigarettes 22
Ecstasy (MDMA) 16, **21**, 29
emotional and stress-related factors 78
emotional development, adolescent developmental arc *74–75*
enabling pattern, behavior argument 12, 41, 46, 48–49, 50, 58, 81
environmental and social factors (prediction, prevention, addressing) 30–35
Erikson, Erik 76
Erlichman, John 35
ethical considerations in HRT practice: autonomy versus paternalism 65; case examples (Jake, Bryan) **68–69**, 69, 125–126; cultural responsiveness 70; ethical dilemmas 58, 63–64, 65; ethical framework and debate 62–65; HRT ethical, legal, and liability challenges 55, 67–69, 149; informed consent 65; mandated substance use treatment 66–67; minor's vs parental rights 66; radical neutrality 57, 64, 149; resource allocation, access to care 65; stigma 65; supervision and training 58
exercises 135–146; (1) harm reduction principles 135; (2) cannabis legalization and harm reduction 135–137; (3) spectrum of adolescent substance use, understanding 137–139; (4) "Walking the Line," safer use continuum with adolescents 139–141; (5) motivational interviewing, mandated client 141–143; (6) parent-teen communication, CRAFT, MI Skills application 144–146

experimental substance use: identity formation, autonomy drive, social influence 76, 78–79; prevalence 22, 23; vs. problematic use differentiation 2–3, 23, 27, 31–32, 45; spectrum of use 90, 137–138, 140; unsafe supply, counterfeit drugs 39; use spectrum 6–7

family and environmental factors 79
family systems theory 2, 71–72, 114, 119, 149
family therapy 2, 31, 49, 87, *124*
fentanyl 16, 39–40, *42*
free play 84
Friedman, J. 39

gateway theory 17, 25–26, 30, 49
Good Samaritan laws 28, 40
Groves, M. 114

Hadland, S. 39
Haidt, Jonathan 84–85
hallucinogens 21, **21**
harm potential, substance use 25–30; adolescent specific symptoms 27–28; gateway theory 25–26, 30; physical 28–29; psychological 29–30
Harm Reduction Coalition *see* National Harm Reduction Coalition's (NHRC)
harm reduction, concept and principles 5, 6–10; community-based/PWUD-including policy creation 8; empowerment, self-determination, peer education/support 8–9; exercise (harm reduction principles) 135; nonjudgement, respect 8; pragmatism, realism (public health framework vs punishment approach) 6; success definition (life quality over abstinence) 7–8; tenets, principles (NHRC) 151; use spectrum acknowledgement 6–7, 7
harm reduction, history 5–6; HIV/AIDS epidemic response 5; international approaches 6; Merseyside heroin approach 5; United States, pre-Harrison Narcotics Act (1914) 6
Harm reduction psychotherapy (Tatarsky) 153
Harm Reduction Therapy (HRT), adolescence adaptability 86–96; addiction as complex biopsychosocial phenomenon 88–90; addiction vs. physical dependence 93–94; drug use spectrum 90–93; dynamic adaptive learning approach 87; family context acknowledgement 87–88; harm reduction tenets 86, 151; reality-based drug education 90; safer use continuum 94–96, **95**
Harm Reduction Therapy (HRT), core dilemmas 60–72; cultural responsiveness needs 44, 69–72, 70, 71, 149; depth vs behavioral focus 61–62; ethical considerations, challenges *see* ethical considerations in HRT practice; initiating vs responding 61; legal considerations, challenges 63, 67, *69–69*; mandated care/treatment *42*, 45, 66–67, 111–112, 141–143; process-content balance 60–61; therapeutic neutrality and engagement 62–63
Harm Reduction Therapy (HRT), in practice 97–114; case example (Brianna) 107–110; Cognitive Behavioral Therapy (CBT) 52, 110, 112, 113–114, 116, 134, 153; Decisional Balance approach 102–104, **104**, 108, 109, 111–112; Dialectical Behavior Therapy (DBT, DBT-A) 52, 110, 114, 116; Drug, Set, Setting model (Zinberg) 51, 52–53, 97–98, 100–102, *100*, 105; Integrated Dynamic Engagement Assessment framework(IDEA) 97, 100, 102, 104–105, 106–110; Motivational Interviewing (MI) *see* Motivational Interviewing (MI); Multidisciplinary Assessment Profile (MAP) 97, **98**, 99, 102; Stages of Change Model (SOC) 47, 53, 67, 105–105, 111, 132, 149
Harm Reduction Therapy (HRT), key considerations 55–59; dialectical nature 55, 57–58, 149; empirical support provision, challenge 58–59; infinite flexibility 56, 149; radical neutrality 56–57, 63, 64, 149; supervision and training 58
Harm Reduction Works (HRW) 44, 154
Harrison Narcotics Act (1914) 6
Hart, Carl 36
hazardous/chaotic substance use 7, 7, 92; environmental and social factors 8, 30–32; harms (personal, family impact) 8, 26, 29, 29–32, 66, 93; physical risks 29, 93; psychological risks 29–30, 93; use spectrum 7, 7, 90, 138–139
Hepatitis B 11, 12
heroin 5, 15, 17, **22**, 24, **24**, 35
Heyman, Gene 88
Hill, M. 37
"hitting bottom" narrative/myth 47–48, 132
HIV 5, 8, 11–12, 13, 14, 15, 148
HRH413 (Harm Reduction Hedgehogs 413) 44, 154
Humanistic Psychology (Maslow) 55

identity formation **75**, 77–78, 81, 97, 149
The Illicit Project 29
The International Conference on the Reduction of Drug Related Harm 6
immigration 71
impulsivity 77, 79, 86, 128, 149
indigenous healing pathways 70
infinite flexibility 56, 149
initiation, age of onset 25–26, 30, 31, 45, 148; *see also* Gateway Theory

Integrated Dynamic Engagement Assessment (IDEA) framework 97, 100, 102, 104–105, 106–110
Integrative Harm Reduction Psychotherapy (IHRP) 52, 115–116
intergenerational trauma 35, 70
International Harm Reduction Coalition 6

Jenkins, E. 33
Johnson Institute Intervention (JII) 120–121
Jones, C. J. 72
"Junkie-Bond," Rotterdam, Netherlands 15
"Just Say No" approach 2, 3, 17, 37

Kandel, Denise 25
Kellogg, Scott 7, 51, 52, 59, 72
Khantzian, Edward 88
Kidorf, M. 12
King, C. 35, 41, 50
Know Drugs program *43*

language and communication impact 16, 49–50, 72
Latine people 46, 70; *see also* racism
Levengood 14
LGBTQ+ 8, 12, 71
Little, Jeannie 51–52, 55–56, 57–58, 60, 94, 97–98, 115, 118–119
Liverpool Drug Dependency Unit (LDDU) 6
LSD 21, **21**
Lukianoff, G. 84

mandated care/treatment *42*, 45, 66–67, 111–112, 141–143
mandated reporting 34, 67, 68
marijuana *see* cannabis
Marlatt, Alan 9, 50
Maslow, Abraham H. 55
Maté, Gabor 88
MDMA 16, **21**, 29
medicalization and disease model narrative *43*, 50, 88–89
mental health 26, 29–30, 32, *42*, 45–46, 76, 89, 92, 101, 124–126
Mersey Drug Training and Information Center (MDTIC) 5–6
Merseyside, UK 5–6
Meyers, Robert J. 81–82, 119–120, 152–153
Miller, William R. 51, 57, 89, 110, 114
Monitoring the Future (MTF) 17–18, 19, 20, 22, 23
Motivational Interviewing (MI) 33, 52, 57, 61, 68; case scenario 111–113; concept, potential 110–111; decisional balance 102–103; example 67; exercises (mandated client, parent-teen communication) 141–143, 144; righting reflex 57

Multi-Dimensional Family Therapy (MDFT) 31
Multidisciplinary Assessment Profile (MAP) 97, **98**, 99, 102
mushrooms 21, **21**, 92

Najavits, Lisa M. 116
naloxone access laws 40, 41
NAMI (National Alliance on Mental Illness) Family Support Groups 128, 130
Narcotics Anonymous (NA) 7–8, *42*, 88
National Epidemiologic Survey on Alcohol and Related Conditions (NESARC) 47
National Harm Reduction Coalition's (NHRC) 5, 6, 86, 151
National Institute on Drug Abuse (NIDA) 12, 19, 88
National Survey on Drug Use and Health (NSDUH) 17, 19, 23–24
The Natural Mind (Weil) 51
needs hierarchy 102, 103–104
neglectful (uninvolved) parenting *80*, 81, 119
Netherlands 12, 15
neutrality, therapeutic 56–57, 62–63, 64, 149
New York 12, 14, 15, 44
nicotine 7, 22, **23**, 76; *see also* tobacco
North American Syringe Exchange Network (NASEW) 12

occasional/sporadic substance use 7, 7, 23, 37, 91, 138
OnPointNYC 14
opiates 12, 13, 14, **22**, 28–29, 61
opioids 16, 24, **24**, 61, 93–94, 101
Over the Influence (Denning and Little) 94
overdose 28–29, 39–40; fatal 28–29, 148; overdose prevention facilities (OPF), centers 13–15, 44, 63, 65, 148; post-treatment overdose 66; prevalence, US 16, 28; prevention education *42*, 57

parental drug use 37
parenting styles: authoritarian *80*, 81; authoritative 44, 73, 74, *80*, 81–83, 84–85, 121, 149; neglectful (uninvolved) *80*, 81, 119; permissive *80*, 81
parents, parenting 3; all use is 27; "all use is abuse," stigmatization approach 3, 16, 30, 38; enabling 46, 48–49, 50; gateway theory 49; hitting bottom 50; initiation, traditional explanation 16; parental drug use, impact 37; problematic vs non-problematic substance use differentiation 27; prohibition-based drug policy, impact on 44–45; punitive-based approach internalizing 24, 34, 46–49; relationship support (communication, monitoring, boundaries) 26, 31; *see also* family systems theory; family therapy; "tough love" concept 44, 46, 48–49, 132, 148

Partnership to End Addiction 154
paternalism 8, 65
Peele, Stanton 81–83, 84, 88
peer influence, education, support 2, 9, 15, 30, 31–34–35, 45–46, 64, 73–*74*, 78, *100*
people of color 9, 44, 66; *see also* racism
permissive parenting *80*, 81
Person-Centered Therapy (Rogers) 55
physical dependence 93–94
physical development, adolescent developmental arc *74–75*
physical risks and harms 28–29, 93
Post, B. C. 70
poverty 9, 46, 101, 118, 119, 135
Practicing Harm Reduction Psychotherapy (Denning and Little) 55
Prescription Drug Abuse Policy System (PDAPS) 40
prescription medication 24, **24**, 39, 40
prescription programs, heroin 15
problematic substance use 7, 7, 92; adolescent specific presentation 27–28; environmental and social factors 9, 30–32, 34, 44; vs. experimental use differentiation 2–3, 23, 27, 31–32, 45; harm potential 27–28, 29; parental use, impact 37; prevalence 23; trauma impact 9, 147; use spectrum 7, 7, 92, 138
prohibition-based policies: criminalization, collateral sanctions 33–34; family/parenting impact 44–45; language and communication impact 16, 49–50; myths 46–49; narrative, theories *42*, 43, 49, 148; narratives and substance use perception/treatment 40–41; school/community impact 16, 29, 44–45; *see also* War on Drugs
psychedelics 35–38, 92
psychological risk factors, harm 29–30; *see also* mental health

racism, racialized stress 9, 70–71, 101, 118, 119, 135, 151
radical neutrality 56–57, 63, 64, 149
Rathus, J. H. 114
RAVE Act 16, 28
regular substance use 7, 7, 91–92; environmental and social factors 30–34; vs. experimental, differentiation 23; harm potential 18; physical, psychological risks 26–30; prevalence of acceptance 18; prevalence of use 18, *18–21*, **21–22**, 26; use spectrum 7, 7, 92, 138
religious and spiritual identity 71
Researching Adolescent Distress and Resilience (RADAR) study 33
resilience, resiliency-based interventions 32–33, 84, 85, 148
Resilient Families initiative, Melbourne, Australia 32–33

righting reflex concept 57
Rigter, H. 31
risk taking behavior 26, 77, 81, 84, 86, 91–92, 149
Robert Wood Johnson Foundation (RWJF) 12
Rogers, Carl R. 55
Rollnick, Stephen 57, 110

Safe Consumption Sites, Safe Injection Facilities 13, 15
safer supply, drug checking 16, 28, 33, 35, 148
safer use continuum 94–96, **95**
Safety First program 36, 37, *43*
San Francisco 8, 13, 15
Satir, Virginia 87
school environment, school programs 32–33, 34–35
school impact of prohibition-based drug policy 45–46
school-family partnership 32–33
school-to-prison pipeline 45–46
Seeking Safety treatment 116–118
SMART Recovery Family & Friends, program and handbook 134, 153–154
social development, adolescent developmental arc *74–75*
social media impact in adolescent development 83–84
Social Media Regulation Act, Utah 84
societal framing of substance use 1–2
spectrum of substance use 3, 6–7, 7, 36, 50, 88, 90–94, 137–139
sporadic/occasional substance use 7, 7, 23, 37, 91, 138
Stages of Change Model (SOC) 47, 53, 67, 105–105, 111, 132, 149
Stanford REACH lab 36
Steinberg, Laurence 73–74, 75–76, 78, 79, 81, 82, 84
Stockwell, T. 27
Strange Situation studies (Ainsworth) 119
Student Assistance Programs (SAPs) 45
Substance Abuse and Mental Health Services Administration (SAMHSA) 19–20, 88, 134
substance use disorder (SUD) 23–24, **23–24**, 27–28, 43, 47, 49, 51, 76, 89, 93–94
supply safety, drug checking 16, 28, 33, 35, 148
Swadi, Harith 31
syringe access, exchange 5–6, 8, 11–13, 14, 35, 148

Tapert, S. F. 27–28
Tatarsky, Andrew 51–52, 59, 72, 115, 153
The Ten Basic Principles of Good Parenting (Steinberg) 81
THC (delta-9-tetrahydrocannabinol) 28–29, 37; *see also* cannabis
tobacco 22–23, **22–24**, 25–26, 28, 33

"tough love" concept 44, 46, 48–49, 132, 148
Toumbourou, J. 33–34
tranquilizers **22**, **24**
Transtheoretical Model 47, 53
trauma: attachment, role in 119; case example (Jason) 127–130; community trauma 35, 70; HRT model 118–119; Integrative Harm Reduction Psychotherapy (IHRP) 115–116; intergenerational 35, 70; racial 70; *Seeking Safety* treatment 116–118; substance vulnerability 9, 30; trauma-informed care 115–119; van der Kolk, bottom-up, bodybased treatments 117–118
Trickett, E. J. 72
Twenge, J. M. 84

uninvolved (neglectful) parenting *80*, 81, 119
Urban Survivor's Union 15
using behavior, trends 17–24; alcohol 20–22, **22**–**23**, 24; cannabis 18, 20, *20*, 23, 27, 90–93; cocaine, crack **22**, **24**, 35, 93, 101–102; Ecstasy (MDMA) **21**; experimental vs. regular or problematic use 23; hallucinogens, LSD 21, **21**; heroin 5, 15, 17, **22**, 24, **24**, 35; opiates **22**; tobacco, nicotine 22–23, **22**–**24**, 25–26, 28, 33; use disorders and treatment 23–24, **23**–**24**; vaping 22–23, **22**–**23**

Vakharia, S. 41, 58–59, 59
van der Kolk, Bessel A. 117–118
Van Sciver, A. 114
Vancouver Area Network of Drug Users (VANDU), Canada 15
vaping 22–23, **22**–**23**, *68*–*69*, 138, 140

Wade, N. G. 71
War on Drugs 2, 6, 35, 39, *41*–*43*, 52, 66, 132, 148
We The Village 152–153
Weil, Andrew 51
Welsh, J. 32
Wicklund, R. A. 45
Witkiewitz, K. 9
World Health Organization (WHO) 6

Zero-Tolerance approaches 2, 34, 44, 45, 132, 148
Zinberg, Norman 51, 52, 97–98, 100–101, *100*, 105

Made in the USA
Monee, IL
03 May 2026

49437540R00103